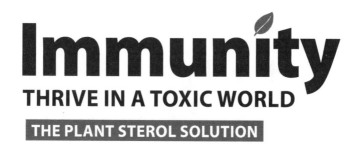

Immunity

THRIVE IN A TOXIC WORLD

THE PLANT STEROL SOLUTION

ALAN FERGUSSON and JACK DAVIDSON

D0962933

ActNatural Corporation
5948 3rd Line RR#1
Hillsburgh, ON
N0B 1Z0

ISBN: 978-0-9867247-3-2

Copy Writing: Healthy Awareness Inc.
Copy Editing: Susan F. Watts, RN, BScN
Book and Cover Design: Jasper van Meurs

Printed in Canada by Friesens Corp.

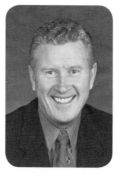 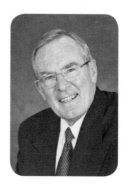

Jack Davidson   Alan Fergusson

The founders of Celt Naturals and
and the developers of Immuno-Care®

"It is gratifying to me as a physician to see quality products enter the market. I know of no other plant sterol product with the health enhancing immune benefits offered by Immuno-Care."

- Dr Allen Tyler, MD., PhD., ND.
  Former medical director of the State of Washington

Contents

🌿 Foreword

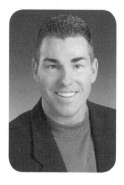

I have noticed many new and exciting changes in the world of alternative medicine. New research has resulted in re-formulation of old natural remedies to achieve even better clinical results. A shift continues in our society as more people explore the option of alternative medicine.

Many practitioners of mainstream medicine are now exploring natural alternatives to fill the gap where drug therapy has failed. People are much better educated and aware of natural alternatives to treat themselves and their families. Naturopathic schools are turning out more doctors than ever before, as more people now demand natural alternatives to drug therapy where possible.

There is a time and a place for everything! The time, place and introduction of Immuno-Care® couldn't be better! Our environment is rapidly changing and so is our health. We eat nutrient-depleted foods that lack the proper nutrition to sustain vibrant health. Our foods are over-processed, pesticides are sprayed on our crops and grains are genetically modified for convenience. We are bombarded by strains of flu never heard of before, colds that linger for weeks or months, and exotic viruses such as SARS and West Nile that compromise our immune systems. We need to protect our health!

I know of no other plant sterol-based product on the market that has the health-enhancing immune benefits offered by Immuno-Care®. It is refreshing to find a supplement that works so well and gives people a chance to reclaim their health.

I trust this product. You should too!

Yours in Abundant Health,

Brad King, MS, MFS

Bestselling author, formulator and researcher
www.AwakenYourBody.com

Acknowledgements ————————

This book is, in a way, a reflection of the many people who have inspired us and taught us that no matter what life presents to us, it can be overcome. We believe that it's not by chance that certain people come into our lives and that we each have something to learn and something to give. These moments can be potential opportunities for growth.

Without the encouragement and support of Deane Parkes, whose longtime association with the 'health industry' and all the knowledge and experience that this encompasses, we simply could not have written this book. His belief in us and in Immuno-Care® prompted us to share our message with others. He continues to encourage people to make lifestyle changes that will enable them to return to health and wellness.

We express our thanks and gratitude to our longtime friend Linda Pedersen. For 11 years, she has believed in us and our product and has never given up supporting us and inspiring us. She has an amazing drive to help people with health issues, and to provide them with hope and with answers.

A special thanks to all the staff at Preferred Nutrition, for welcoming us into your family. Your guidance and friendship has been invaluable.

Our appreciation to Dr. Ludo Brunel, Brad King and Julie Daniluk for their contributions to this book, which we are sure readers will find informative and helpful.

A special thanks to Gifford-Jones MD for his support, interest in the product.

Our thanks to Lisa Petty for her patience and help in getting the draft information printer ready, and to the countless others who have lent their support.

For the staff in all the health food stores and practitioners who have joined with us in the quest to help others seek a healthier lifestyle over the years, we are most grateful.

Finally, to all those who have shared their stories with us and allowed us to be part of their journey towards health, we offer a sincere "Thank you."

Alan & Jack

The Importance of Plant Sterols in a Toxic World

by Dr. Ludo Brunel ND.

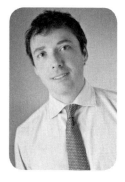

Every day we are exposed to innumerable toxins and chemicals in the environment that can cause serious damage to our bodies and to our health. These toxins can be significant contributors to the development of many chronic diseases, including cancer and heart disease. From pesticides and herbicides to exhaust fumes to heavy metals in the foods we eat, it is impossible to avoid exposure to these hazardous substances.

Once inside our bodies, toxic chemicals damage our cells and DNA, and weaken the immune system. In *Immunity – Thrive in a Toxic World*, Jack Davidson and Alan Fergusson explain how this is especially detrimental, given that the immune system is an essential line of defence against the very toxins we encounter daily. But the immune system is also meant to detect invaders and protects us against the damage they can cause. Unfortunately, constant exposure to toxins can throw this highly tuned system out of balance, leading to greater and more serious health problems. For example, the immune system's reaction to injury is inflammation – a normal response that is part of the healing process. Constant exposure to irritating and damaging toxins, however, can cause continual stimulation of this response, leading to chronic inflammation. Chronic inflammation is a serious condition, linked to many diseases. In addition to this, continual exposure to toxins can exhaust the body's antioxidant supplies, leading to free radical damage and cell injury. The overall effect, in which some parts of the immune system are overactive and some are suppressed, results in a state of imbalance in the body's immune response. In turn, this leads to an increased susceptibility to disease, an increased risk of auto-immune disorders and a reduced ability to fight infections.

It is clear that maintaining a strong immune system is essential for supporting health in a toxic world. But that is not the end of the story. In this book, you will learn that an immune response that spins out of control is also dangerous to health. The key is balance. Research has shown that a type of fat or 'sterol' found in plants plays a very important role in achieving this balance.

Plant sterols also mediate some of the effects that can result from constant exposure to toxins in the environment. These fats are similar in structure to cholesterol, but do not have the negative effects usually associated with cholesterol. In fact, plant sterols are well known for their benefits in helping to reduce cholesterol levels in humans.

Plant sterols are unique to plants and cannot be made by the human body. As such, they must be obtained from our food or from nutritional supplements. While plant sterols are naturally found in many of the plant-based foods we eat, they are present in small quantities, making it difficult to obtain beneficial doses from the diet alone. This is especially true given that modern processing and storage methods significantly deplete the nutrient and sterol content of our foods. Therefore, daily supplementation can be very helpful for achieving an optimal dose of the right kinds of plant sterols to support a healthy immune system.

Plant sterols are a superior choice to other immune system support products: many other products act only to stimulate the immune response and should be taken for short periods of time. Plant sterols act to balance the immune system, making them well-suited for everyday use.

Researchers studied plant sterols for several conditions, including tuberculosis (a bacterial infection), rheumatoid arthritis (an auto-immune condition where the body's immune system over-reacts and begins attacking its own tissues) and immune suppression in marathon runners following intense exercise. In all cases, plant sterols provided a beneficial effect on the immune system, helping to improve and balance the response, relieving symptoms and reducing inflammation.

Overall, research shows that daily intake of plant sterols can help to reduce immune suppression associated with stressful or toxic conditions and also to protect against excessive inflammation and damage that occurs as a result of these same conditions. This, in turn, can help to protect the body from damage and reduce the risk of future health problems and disease.

Immunity – Thrive in a Toxic World reveals that a balanced immune system is a healthy immune system, and plant sterols are an effective way to help you achieve this balance.

PART ONE: Introduction

CHAPTER **ONE**

Stacking the Odds

Jack Davidson and Alan Fergusson are two men with a strong message. They believe that exercise, a positive attitude, and a supplement called Immuno-Care® are three critical components for a healthy immune system.

Many years ago, Alan was providing support to a man with prostate cancer. At the time, he said that he wished that he had explored alternatives to the traditional medical treatments. These words came back with a vengeance when, several years later, Alan found himself facing a similar problem: elevated prostate-specific antigen (PSA) levels. PSA is a protein produced by cells of the prostate gland. The higher a man's PSA level, the more likely the risk of cancer being present. Consequently, Alan became strongly motivated to explore alternative ways of dealing with the situation.

Jack has always had an interest in health and fitness. In fact, as a teenager he won several championships as a long distance runner, an interest he continued to pursue as an adult. He suffered from severe allergies, however, and would say that he hated the first signs of spring because he knew that allergy season was just around the corner. Within minutes of passing a ditch filled with weeds or grasses, his eyes would swell, and along would come the runny nose and achy joints. This was not only a condition that afflicted him during his leisure hours; it could surface in a business environment as Jack, to his embarrassment, found out when undergoing an important interview.

Natural defense

As the body comes with a very well-designed system for defense and healing, Alan and Jack decided to focus on the immune system. After considerable research, they discovered that plant sterols can inhibit the growth of breast, colon and prostate cancer cells. In fact, sterols had been used in Germany for over 20 years for the relief of benign prostatic hyperplasia (BPH), a condition frequently occurring in older men where they have difficulty urinating due to inflammation of the prostate. Perhaps even more astounding was the fact that research had shown that beta-sitosterol (the active sterol in the phytosterol mixture) could not only inhibit the growth of cancer cells, but it could also increase the rate at which cancer cells die.

However, sterols are easily destroyed by acids in the stomach and not readily absorbed by the body. So it was critical to discover a way to not only protect the sterols from stomach acids, but also to facilitate their absorption.

Immuno-Care® is born

Researching the sterols and their absorption was the first step. The second step was to reduce the risk for the development of further cancers from free radicals within the body (since these can damage DNA) by identifying a broad-spectrum antioxidant.

Then the researchers had to ensure that the components worked together and were also bio-available to the body – meaning that the body could absorb and use them. Their efforts paid off: no other product had this synergistic combination. Few products have the distinction of being awarded a patent, and Immuno-Care® is one of them.

Now, several years later, Alan's PSA levels have dropped substantially. Originally developed for Alan, the combination of natural ingredients in Immuno-Care® have been shown to have a remarkable capacity to alleviate many of the symptoms related to immune system disorders, such as fibromyalgia, psoriasis, asthma, chronic fatigue syndrome and rheumatoid arthritis, as well as many allergies, common colds and flu.

With the escalating introduction of viruses such as the West Nile and SARS, it is becoming increasingly important to maintain a strong immune system. It is a supplement that people can take on a daily basis to maintain their body's ability to fight disease in general, and in particular, to reduce the potential risk of breast, colon and prostate cancers.

What is unique about this story is that during their research, Jack and Alan found that people with mul-

Jack says, "It was such a relief to me when we discovered that Immuno-Care® could play a significant role in alleviating the symptoms associated with allergies. Not long after starting the product, my allergies were gone. To this day, it is rare that I experience an allergic reaction, and if I do then I take a larger dose of Immuno-Care®. Within a few hours, the symptoms subside. Immuno-Care® has been a Godsend for me."

tiple personalities show symptoms of illness that occur and disappear with changes in their personality. This led Jack and Alan to believe that there is a very important psychological/spiritual component to healing that leads to peace of mind, which is just as important as diet, exercise and supplements. Unfortunately, this component is frequently ignored, perhaps because it involves what is often a very difficult internal journey.

"Healing is not just a matter of taking two pills a day," says Alan. "It is an internal journey that involves changes of both attitude and perception, which is why it is so difficult. The program that I developed for myself to address this very important area is outlined below. This is a program that helped me, but someone else would have to adapt it to meet their own specific situation. At least it is a starting point."

All kidding aside
Now that he is no longer bothered by summer allergies, Jack has to mow the lawn and do other garden chores. He jokes, "There is a dark side to every discovery! I wouldn't change it for the world, though. For years, I was unable to enjoy the outdoors to the extent that I do now. Life is so much more enjoyable".

Although Immuno-Care® was originally developed to help battle cancer, Jack and Alan emphasize Immuno-Care® is not a cure for cancer. It is, however, something that can help you "stack the odds" in your favour. Their philosophy is that dealing with cancer, or any other serious condition, is a matter of trying to change the odds in your favour, using all the resources available: traditional and alternative, physical and spiritual. It starts when you take control.

The road of alternative treatments is a road much less travelled, but more and more people are finding it worth exploring. It is amazing how many people facing serious illnesses show signs of improvement once they start to become proactive and take control of their own health.

Alan's Healthy Living Program

Here are some of the changes that Alan incorporated into his life. You will have to adapt these to meet your own needs, but at least it is a starting point. May you find joy and peace on your healing journey.

- Live one day (and sometimes one minute) at a time. Try to enjoy each day. Leave yesterday's mistakes where they belong: in yesterday. They are yesterday's rain showers.

- Exercise regularly. Alan chose running. He ran his first 8K road race in Victoria in 1993 and, until recently, ran or swam most days to keep fit. (Alan is now 78 years old.)

- Give positive messages to yourself, and particularly to your body. It is probably your best friend; don't be afraid to give it a hug and say thanks. Think more about sunsets, music, love and laughter.

- Remember why you are here, where you came from, and where you are going. Life is only an interlude.

- Remember that you are 'perfectly imperfect.' You came designed the way you are. So don't be surprised when you screw up; it's an opportunity for learning and for growth, for both yourself and any other party involved.

- Assign time for prayer/meditation: spend more time listening than asking.

- Identify your needs, touch more people and reach out for help. Remember, it generally takes more grace to receive than it does to give.

- Practice visualizing/imaging on a regular basis.

- Join a therapy/support group, but make sure it provides positive support. You may be surprised to find that you are not the only one who sometimes feels that you are in a psychological tumbler dryer, and that it is okay to feel that way.

- Banish the word *should* and replace it with *could*. Never again let anyone *should* on you. You steer your own ship.

To explore this road further, read *Peace, Love, and Healing* by Bernie Siegel, MD. It is available through most bookstores for approximately $20 for the soft cover edition, and may be one of the best investments you or someone you love can make if facing a serious illness.

CHAPTER **TWO**
Some Immune Systems Need Help

Let's jump right in and say that your body is the most amazing machine ever built! The human body is highly adaptive, more so than any robot or computer will ever be. No man-made system can be compared to the human body in its inherent complexity and perfection.

The human body is a very vulnerable organism, except for the very strong line of defense that the immune system has thrown around it. Without the natural defense system provided by the immune system, the body would decompose within a few days as a result of bacteria, microbes, viruses, toxins, and parasites. That is what happens when the body dies and the immune system is no longer there. The human immune system works 24/7, though its work never comes to the limelight. The failure of the immune system, however, is easily noticeable.

Although we inhale and ingest thousands of germs every day, the immune system prevents them from causing diseases. If a germ breaks through this preventive barrier, we become ill. Once the immune system discovers these germs, it fights them. If successful, we get over the malady.

Amazing facts about your body:

- You lose approximately 50 to 100 hairs from your head every day, but they are replaced that same day.
- Most people drink 16,000 gallons of water in their lifetime.
- Around 45 miles of nerves run through our body. These electrical impulses travel at a speed of almost 250 mph.
- By age 70, your heart has beaten 2.5 million times and pumped approximately 48 million gallons of blood.
- In a tiny drop of blood, there are 5 million red blood cells, 10,000 white cells and 300,000 platelets.
- One square inch of human skin contains 20 feet of blood vessels, 100 sweat glands and 3 million cells.
- The average human body contains enough: sulfur to kill all the fleas on an average dog, carbon to make 900 pencils, potassium to fire a toy cannon, fat to make 7 bars of soap, phosphorus to make 2,200 match heads and water to fill a ten gallon tank.
- You produce a quart of saliva daily: 10,000 gallons in a lifetime.
- A square inch of human skin has 32 million bacteria on it
- Each second, 10 million cells die and are replaced in your body.
- You create new skin over your entire body every month and a new skeleton every 3 months.
- Your ears and nose don't stop growing during your entire lifetime.

The major parts of the immune system are the thymus, spleen, lymph system, bone marrow, white blood cells, antibodies, complement system, and hormones. The immune system is made up of a network of cells, tissues and organs that work together to protect the body. The cells involved are white blood cells, or leukocytes, which come in two basic types that combine to seek out and destroy disease-causing organisms and substances.

Immune System Facts:

The first layers of our bodies are the skin and mucous membranes, which act as the physical barrier to harmful organisms and substances. The second protective layer is the 'innate immune system.' It acts as a short-term non-specific immune response. If the first and second protective barriers are crossed by the microbes, the invaders encounter the third and more active immune response. (When the immune system attacks a harmless substance or chemical in the body, it leads to an allergic reaction. We'll discuss allergies in greater detail in coming pages.)

Factors affecting immune health:

- The environment plays an important role in affecting our immune response.
- Toxic substances, air pollution, pesticides and second-hand cigarette smoke affect the defense system of our body.
- It is very important to get your beauty sleep for at least 8 hours; less than 5 hours sleep can significantly depress your immune functions.
- You may lose five billion white blood cells when donating blood and still be left with enough to fight a full-fledged immune response.
- Too much of anything can be harmful. Similarly, some sunlight helps the body produce vitamin D and too much sunlight suppresses the immune system.

Research shows that many diseases stem from a poor functioning immune system. In theory, it has so many built-in fail-safes that we should rarely fall ill. But, in fact, we do. The system can simply be overwhelmed by the number and toxicity of viruses, bacteria or other foreign cells and toxins. Add toxins that the immune system must investigate and control as necessary (herbicides, pesticides, food additives) and it's easy to imagine the impact all this has on the immune response. Then, throw in the immense amount of radiation from depletion of the ozone layer, plus cell phones and TV transmissions and other forms of electropollution that are a common part of life today, and there is a cocktail of nasty events targeting the immune system.

Age, stress, and poor nutrition can sap our immune system of its effectiveness. Influenza provides one example. During young adulthood when the body can mount a robust immune response to this common virus, influenza is rarely fatal. Among the elderly, however, the virus is associated with significant rates of death and hospitalization.[1]

The impact of aging on the immune system is profound. As people age, a number of critical immune system components are reduced or slowed, including cellular response, response to vaccines and antibody production. At the same time, susceptibilities to infection and cancer increase. Some of this increased susceptibility to disease is linked to chronic inflammation, which is associated with many disorders of aging.[2] Age, however, isn't the sole culprit in reduced immune function. There is no question that exercise, stress, and nutritional status play an important role in maintaining a healthy immune system.

> If everyone would take one capsule of Immuno-Care® per day, we would have fewer people suffering from immune-related disorders. If you take care of your health and do a little daily maintenance then it will take care of you!
>
> *Dr Chris Rolston, Edmonton, AB*

Consider just a few of the research findings:

- Dietary deficiencies and malabsorption alter metabolism and exacerbate chronic disorders. An imbalance in the intake of dietary fat, carbohydrate, and protein can contribute to the development of diseases. [3]
- There is overwhelming evidence of the benefits of a good diet on reducing the risk of many chronic diseases. [4]
- Malnutrition causes a decline in immune function and increased susceptibility to infection. [5,6] Likewise, a vitamin or mineral deficiency can suppress immune system function. [6]
- Correct choices of supplements, vitamins, minerals, fatty acids, probiotics and botanicals have been shown to boost immunity and may also reduce the risk of diseases in healthy individuals. [7]
- Psychological health influences the immune system and the course of many diseases. [8] Depression, stress, and anxiety increase the production of pro-inflammatory chemicals in the blood, which in turn can compromise, depress, or suppress the immune system. [9,10,11]
- High levels of anxiety are associated with decreased immune function. [8,12]
- Chronic stress can provoke long-term increases in pro-inflammatory chemicals. For example, care-giving for a relative with a serious medical condition results in long-term immune suppression among women. [13]

We believe that, as we age, it is wise for people to take preventative action to bolster their immune system. This means reducing negative psychological stress, following a physician-approved moderate long-term exercise program, and following a diet including nutrients that have been shown to enhance the immune response and promote health.

The immune system: how it works

The immune system is an elegant and complex set of components that combine to fight disease, infections, and various pathogens. A healthy immune response identifies pathogens as 'non-self' and rapidly destroys them. A depressed immune system, by contrast, will allow invading organisms to flourish. On the other hand, when the immune system mistakenly recognizes a 'self' cell as a 'non-self' and mounts an immune response, the result is an autoimmune disorder such as allergies or rheumatoid arthritis.

In general, the body has two primary defense mechanisms: natural immunity and acquired immunity. Natural immunity is the 'first responder' to an attack. The natural immune response relies on various white blood cells and physical barriers to block or immediately attack any foreign invader and attempt to destroy it.

These natural defenses include the following organs, chemicals and processes. The first lines of defense are the skin and mucous membranes. Skin forms a physical barrier that prevents most pathogens from entering the body. Glands in the skin secrete lactic acid and fatty acid, which make the skin surface acidic, preventing bacterial growth. The outer layer of skin flakes off, which removes bacteria and prevents the entrance of many pathogens. There are many secondary barriers. For example, tears, sweat, and saliva combat some bacteria. The hydrochloric acid and protein-digesting enzymes secreted by the stomach are lethal to many, but not all, pathogens.[14]

Acquired immunity, on the other hand, involves antibodies that are created in response to specific foreign antigens. This sort of response requires a few days for the body to recognize the invader and manufacture antibodies against it. Once the body has manufactured a particular antibody for a specific invader, the immune system response is faster and more effective should that invader appear again. [1,14]

Inflammation is a nonspecific response to infection or tissue injury; inflammation is one of the initial responses to the presence of an invader and focuses the immune system at the site of infection. Inflammation draws phagocytes, which attack and kill the invading microbe and interact with the adaptive immune system to create a long-term response. It can also cause considerable damage to host tissues, however, which can be part of the microbial pathogenesis of a disease process. In addition, unwanted inflammation can be a major destructive force, as seen in many autoimmune diseases. The four signs of the inflammatory response are redness, swelling, heat, and pain. Inflammation begins when the cells release certain cytokines, including interleukins (IL-1 and IL- 6), and tumour necrosis factor-alpha (TNF-alpha). [14]

Phagocytic cells engulf foreign cells and destroy pathogens. The phagocytic cells are white blood cells and include neutrophils, eosinophils, and macrophages; they have short lives and must be carefully replenished by the body. Neutrophils and macrophages are a very important aspect of the natural or innate defenses of the body. [14] The innate immune system is nonspecific as to the type of organism it fights and is ready to be mobilized upon the first signs of infection.

Natural killer (NK) cells destroy certain cancer cells and a variety of pathogens. Killer cells are active secretors of interferon, an important

> Laughter is the best medicine. This is not just an old saying, but laughter induces a proactive immune response that leads to a healthy body!

potent protein that modulates the response of the immune system. Natural killer cells attach directly to the surfaces of infected cells and cause them to burst. They can also kill a pathogen by making its outer membrane leak.[14]

Our cells use chemicals to communicate with one another, with each chemical sending a different message. These chemical messengers are called cytokines. Cytokines regulate immunity, inflammation, and the production of white blood cells. There are dozens of cytokines, and each performs a specific set of activities against target cells. They can act in concert or in opposition.

Nutrition, immunity, and your genes

Have you ever noticed how some people seem never to get sick, but others are constantly battling colds and the flu? Researchers are just now beginning to understand how genes affect nutrition and overall immunity.

It turns out that overall risk of contracting many diseases is influenced by genetics.[15] A new field called nutritional genomics explores the interaction of nutrition, genes, and environmental factors, including diet.[3] While the field is relatively new, a well-studied example of the relationship between genetics and diet is type 2 diabetes. This condition is associated with a sedentary lifestyle, being overweight, and ethnicity. Although some individuals are genetically predisposed to diabetes, many can control symptoms through exercise and a change in diet.[3] In the future, genetic testing might be able to help physicians recommend specific, personal nutritional programs that are tailored to each individual's unique genetic makeup and that will help us fight disease and stay healthy. Stay tuned for more exciting and useful discoveries in the field of nutrigenomics.

Support your healthy immune system

Keeping the immune system in proper working order, especially with the increasing amounts of toxic pollutants we are exposed to in the environment, is becoming a tough task. Many physicians are now concerned about 'super bugs' and research experts and medical professionals agree that a strong immune system is critical to staying healthy.

A healthy immune system grows ever more important as we age, and immune status is closely associated with nutrition, exercise, and stress reduction. Older people and people with compromised immune systems are advised to talk to their physician about exercising, reducing stress and designing an active, immune-boosting nutritional program.

Along with familiar nutrients (vitamins, minerals, healthy fats), antioxidants, plant sterols and phytonutrients play a vital role in helping to support the immune system. Let's explore each of them in turn.

Antioxidants

You may have heard about the health benefits of antioxidants, but do you know what they are and how they actually work?

Antioxidants help fight oxidation, a normal chemical process that takes place in the body every day. It's much like the chemical reaction that creates rust on a bicycle

I really appreciate you sending me Immuno-Care® in the mail. I am certainly a faithful believer in your product. I am a nurse and work with very sick people every day. I find that if I do feel something coming on, it is short-lived using Immuno-Care®.

N.P., Kingston ON

or turns the surface of a cut apple brown. Oxidation can be accelerated by stress, cigarette smoking, and alcohol. When there are disruptions in the natural oxidation process, highly unstable and potentially damaging molecules called free radicals are created. Oxygen triggers the formation of these destructive little chemicals, and, if left uncontrolled, they can cause damage to cells in the body.

Antioxidants are the knights in shining armour that subjugate the attack of free radicals in the body. Though antioxidants are produced naturally in the body, they decline with age; hence, there is an increasing need to acquire them from our diet. Antioxidants work by neutralizing free radicals that can lead to cell dysfunction and the onset of problems like heart disease and diabetes. Antioxidants may also improve the immune function and perhaps lower your risk of infection and cancer.

Free radicals explained

Free radicals are unstable molecules that readily react with other molecules, especially oxygen, to change their chemical composition. Technically, they are atoms or groups of atoms that contain an odd number of electrons. They can be formed when certain molecules interact with oxygen. Once formed, free radicals want to find another electron to even out their numbers again. This starts a chain of damaging chemical reactions, wherein free radicals steal electrons from other atoms. The biggest danger to the human body is their potential to react with cellular components like DNA or the cell membrane, causing cells to function poorly or die.

Free radicals are not only naturally generated by your body, but they are also present in foods you eat as well as in the air you breathe. Some even come through exposure to sunlight that can harm the eyes and the skin. Free radicals can trap damaging low-density lipoprotein (LDL) in an artery wall and begin the formation of plaque; they can damage DNA; or they can change the course of what enters and leaves a cell. Any of these actions can be the start of a disease process.

Free radical production is actually a normal part of life, part of the equation of simply breathing in oxygen. Usually, the body's natural defense systems neutralize free radicals that develop, rendering them harmless. However, environmental assaults on the body, such as UV-radiation, pollutants and alcohol, can overpower the body's ability to neutralize free radicals, allowing them to cause damage to the structure and function of the body's cells. There is good evidence that this damage contributes to aging and leads

I am writing to thank you for your excellent Immuno-Care® product. It does what it claims and more. While I was undergoing a course of radiation and chemo, I decided to take your product in order to improve my immune system. A side effect of my treatments has been a lymphedema of one of my arms. This summer, I was bitten by mosquitoes on the affected arm. None of the bites became infected, and I am sure that was due to the maintenance of my immune system with Immuno-Care®. Immuno-Care® has enabled me to maintain my health and return to work as a nurse. I noticed that while most of my colleagues went down with seasonal colds and flu, I managed to avoid them. I am so grateful for the friend who recommended Immuno-Care® in the first place.

E., BA Hons RN, Calgary, AB

to a host of illnesses, including cancer and heart disease.

How antioxidants work:

Chain-breaking

When a free radical releases or steals an electron, a second radical is formed. This molecule then turns around and does the same thing to a third molecule, continuing to generate more unstable products. The process continues until termination occurs: either the radical is stabilized by a chain-breaking antioxidant such as beta-carotene and vitamins C and E, or it simply decays into a harmless product.

Preventive

Antioxidant enzymes like superoxide dismutase, catalase and glutathione peroxidase prevent oxidation by reducing the rate of chain initiation. That is, by scavenging initiating radicals, such antioxidants can thwart an oxidation chain from ever getting set in motion. They can also prevent oxidation by stabilizing transition metal radicals such as copper and iron.

The antioxidant process

Antioxidants block the process of oxidation by neutralizing free radicals. In effect, they give up part of themselves and, in doing so, the antioxidants themselves become oxidized. That is why there is a constant need to replenish our antioxidant resources.

The effectiveness of any given antioxidant in the body depends on which free radical is involved, how and where it is generated, and where the target of damage is. Thus, while in one particular system an antioxidant may protect against free radicals, in other systems it could have no effect at all. Or, in certain circumstances, an antioxidant may even act as a *pro-oxidant* that generates toxic oxygen species.

Plant Sterols

One of the most amazing developments in the area of natural remedies is plant sterols, commonly referred to as plant fats. They are described in molecular terms as 'steroidal alcohols.' Sterols occur naturally in the cells and membranes of most plants, seeds, grains, and nuts. The most familiar type of animal sterol is cholesterol. Cholesterol is vital to cellular function, and a precursor to fat-soluble vitamins and steroid hormones.

First discovered in South Africa and used by Zulu tribesmen for generations, plant sterols have been shown to be very beneficial in supporting the immune system. They have been extensively tested in clinical trials involving over 25,000 patients with no known toxicity and no known drug interactions. The best known members of this phytonutrient family are beta-sitosterol, stigmasterol, campesterol, brassicasterol and their associated glucosides. The most remarkable member of this family is beta-sitosterol.

Beta-sitosterol is chemically similar to cholesterol, but is totally different in its biological function. There are litreally hundreds of studies and reports that attest to the effectiveness of beta-sitosterol in preventing disease and maintaining health.

Today's diets are generally deficient

For generations, Sangomas, the traditional healers of Africa, have used herbs to heal and cure the sick. They have knowledge of herbal medicines that help prevent arthritis, heart disease, cancer and many modern day illnesses.

in plant sterols, due to processing and storage methods used in modern food production. Our bodies cannot make plant sterols, and insufficient dietary intake can result in a weak immune system and a consequent deterioration of health.

Phytonutrients:

From the ancient Greek, *phyto* means plant; thus, phytonutrients are plant nutrients. In their natural state, phytonutrients are often bound to the fibres of plants, making them difficult to absorb during digestion, particularly in the case of older people and those having weak digestive systems. Even though their absorption efficiency is low, their apparent synergistic stimulatory effect on the immune system and prophylactic effect on a variety of diseases indicate their importance in human and animal nutrition.

Studies over the past decade have shown phytonutrients to be a valuable adjunct to the prevention and treatment of a wide range of immune-related disorders.

- Phytonutrients can both stimulate an underperforming immune system so that our bodies can combat disease more effectively and can calm down an over-active immune system, as in the autoimmune disorders like rheumatoid arthritis, psoriasis, eczema and CFS.

- Phytonutrients are believed to be one of the few natural, non-toxic substances to safely activate the body's T-cells which control the immune system's response to infection and altered cells like cancer.

- Phytonutrients do not cure disease directly by themselves but rather boost the body's disease-fighting mechanism to enable it to overcome disease naturally. (Many conventional treatments such as anti-inflammatory compounds and immunosuppressive treatments curb the immune system and therefore leave the patient vulnerable to carcinogens and opportunistic infections.)

• Phytonutrients enjoy a major advantage over substances commonly used in the treatment of anti-viral diseases because their function is to maintain and improve the immune system. Their efficacy is not reduced by the evolution of viral resistance, as is the case in other anti-viral treatments.

Unfortunately, modern diets are lacking in sterols. This is partly due to modern processing methods, and because the fat and cholesterol content of these diets tends to inhibit sterol absorption. In the coming pages, we'll address how to make up for these deficiencies.

---

[1] Nichol KL *et al.* Effectiveness of Influenza Vaccine in the Community-Dwelling Elderly. *N Engl J Med.* 2007 357:1373-1381.

[2] Ershler WB, Keller ET. Age-associated increased interleukin-6 gene expression, late-life diseases, and frailty. *Annu Rev Med.* 2000 51:245-2703.

[3] Kaput J, Rodriguez RL. Nutritional genomics: the next frontier in the postgenomic era. *Physiol Genomics.* 2004 Jan 15;16(2):166–77.

[4] Ames BN. DNA damage from micronutrient deficiencies is likely to be a major cause of cancer. *Mutat Res.* 2001 Apr 18;475(1–2):7–20.

[5] Brussow H, Sidoti J *et al.* Effect of malnutrition in Ecuadorian children on titers of serum antibodies to various microbial antigens. *Clin Diag Lab Immunol.* 1995 (2):62–8.

[6] De la Fuente M, Ferrandez M *et al.* Immune function in aged women is improved by ingestion of vitamins C and E. *Can J Physiol Pharmacol.* 1998 (76):373–80.

[7] Kaminogawa S, Nanno M. Modulation of Immune Functions by Foods. *Evid Based Complement Alternat Med.* 2004. Dec 1(3):241-250.

[8] Kiecolt-Glaser J *et al.* Psychoneuroimmunology and psychosomatic medicine: back to the future. *Psychosom Med.* 2000 (641):15–28.

[9] Appels A et al. Inflammation, depressive symptomtology, and coronary artery disease. *Psychosom Med.* 2000 Sep 62(5):601–5.

[10] Dentino AN et al. Association of interleukin-6 and other biologic variables with depression in older people living in the community. *J Am Geriatr Soc.* 1999 Jan 47(1):6–11.

[11] Maes M et al. Elevated serum interleukin-6 (IL-6) and IL-6 receptor concentrations in posttraumatic stress disorder following accidental man-made traumatic events. *Biol Psychiatry.* 1999 Apr 1;45(7):833–9.

[12] Koh KB et al. Reduced lymphocyte proliferation and interleukin-2 production in anxiety disorders. *Psychosom Med.* 1998 Jul 60(4):479–83.

[13] Lutgendorf SK et al. Life stress, mood disturbance, and elevated interleukin-6 in healthy older women. *J Gerontol A Biol Sci Med Sci.* 1999 Sep 54(9): M434–M439.

[14] Janeway CA et al. *Immunobiology: The Immune System in Health and Disease.* London, UK. Garland Publishing. 1999.

[15] Mathew C. Postgenomic technologies: hunting the genes for common disorders. *BMJ.* 2001 Apr 322:1031–4.

CHAPTER **THREE**

✐ Stress and the Mind/Body Connection ──────

Modern life is full of hassles, deadlines, frustrations, and demands. For many people, stress is so commonplace that it has become a way of life. Stress isn't always bad. In small doses, it can help you perform under pressure and motivate you to do your best. But when you're constantly running in emergency mode, your mind and body pay the price.

If you frequently find yourself feeling frazzled and overwhelmed, it's time to take action to bring your nervous system back into balance. You can protect yourself by learning how to recognize the signs and symptoms of stress and taking steps to reduce its harmful effects.

The body's stress response
When you perceive a threat, your nervous system responds by releasing a flood of stress hormones, including adrenaline and cortisol. These hormones rouse the body for emergency action. Your heart pounds faster, muscles tighten, blood pressure rises, breath quickens, and your senses become sharper. These physical changes increase your strength and stamina, speed your reaction

time, and enhance your focus – preparing you to either fight or flee from the danger at hand.

Stress is a normal physical response to events that make you feel threatened or upset your balance in some way. When you sense danger – whether it's real or imagined – the body's defenses kick into high gear in a rapid, automatic process known as the 'fight-or-flight' reaction, or the *stress response.*

The stress response is the body's way of protecting you. When working properly, it helps you stay focused, energetic, and alert. In emergency situations, stress can save your life – giving you extra strength to defend yourself, for example, or spurring you to slam on the brakes to avoid an accident.

The stress response also helps you rise to meet challenges. Stress is what keeps you on your toes during a presentation at work, sharpens your concentration when you're attempting the game-winning free throw, or drives you to study for an exam when you'd rather be watching TV. But beyond a certain point, stress stops being helpful and starts causing major damage to your health, your mood, your productivity, your relationships, and your quality of life.

How do you respond to stress?
It's important to learn how to recognize when your stress levels are out of control. The most dangerous thing about stress is how easily it can creep up on you. You get used to it. It starts to feel familiar, even normal. You don't notice how much it's affecting you, even as it takes a heavy toll.

The signs and symptoms of stress overload can be almost anything. Stress affects the mind, body, and behaviour in many ways, and everyone experiences stress differently.

Too much stress? Signs include:
- Tiring more easily
- Working harder but accomplishing less
- Difficulty finding the joy in life
- Trouble sleeping
- Waking feeling unrested
- Shortness of breath
- Heart palpitations
- Neck or shoulder tension
- Frequent headaches
- Short temper
- Digestion problems

The mind/body connection

Who in North America isn't stressed these days? And when you think of it, stress contributes or is directly associated to most, if not all illness. In our society, many of us are consumed by the overwhelming stress of daily living – from work, school, and/or family demands. Stress, as a result of a fast-paced lifestyle, contributes to physical and psychological distress and illness.

Research shows that psychological stress is associated with several health conditions, such as immune dysfunction, hypertension, gastrointestinal disorders, chronic pain, and cancer, to name a few. Stress is also linked to psychological disorders such as depression and anxiety, which can be then exacerbated with increased stress in one's life. There is a correlation between stress and the psychological effect on health.

One of the things that I learned early on in this journey was that the mind could have an incredible impact on the body. This is clearly illustrated in the following examples:

I remember speaking with a doctor in Phoenix about this same subject and he related a story about a patient who changed personalities during a consultation. The fascinating thing was that the patient was 'hale and hearty' in the first personality but with the second personality, he had a musculoskeletal disorder. The doctor watched the patient change in appearance before his very eyes!

In his book, *Quantum Healing*, Deepak Chopra recites the case of a patient with multiple personalities: in one personality he was diabetic, but when he changed personalities, his blood sugars returned to normal. In another personality, he was allergic to orange juice and would break out in hives; yet, when he changed personalities again, the hives just disappeared! This was the same body!

Bernie Siegel, in his book *Peace, Love and Healing*, tells of a patient who had to sleep with several pairs of glasses by her bedside because she was never sure in which personality she would awaken, and each personality required a different prescription!

Stress and immunity

Research shows that cortisol, a hormone associated with stress, inhibits the proliferative response in the autologous mixed lymphocyte reaction: in everyday language, this means that stress is suppressing your immune system – just when you need it operating at maximum effectiveness![1]

To illustrate how big an impact stress can have, consider a couple of studies quoted by researcher Ronald Glasser in his paper, *Stress-associated Immune Dysregulation.*[2] In one study, a group of healthy senior citizens was taught to practice progressive relaxation and guided imagery. A control group met at the same time, and discussed whatever they wished. After a month, the group practicing visualisation and guided imagery had a 30% enhancement of NK cell activity, which persisted over the next month. Please note that 30% is a very significant increase.

Another study was based on women providing care for a spouse with Alzheimer's disease or dementia, versus a control group. All subjects underwent a 3.5 mm punch biopsy wound at the same site on their bodies. It was found that wounds in caregivers took 24% longer to heal when compared to well-matched control subjects. Or to put it another way, the non-caregivers, who would be less stressed than the caregivers, healed 24% faster than the stressed caregivers.

Likewise, in another study of dental students who volunteered to receive oral punch biopsies, healing took 40% longer during examination periods than during summer vacation, with no student showing faster healing during exams than during vacation. [3]

Need more convincing about the mind/body relationship and how it relates to stress and immunity? You are invited to read some of the research published in peer-reviewed journals and listed for you at the end of the chapter. If you're skeptical: don't feel bad. I (Alan) was, too, at one time! [11-19]

The stress of illness

These days, many people are being diagnosed with cancer, which is a common cause of stress. When undergoing a diagnosis or treatment for a disease, much of the stress seems to arise from a sense of helplessness and despair, and I (Alan) can certainly attest to this. Getting poked and punctured, then waiting for the results. And then there are the worries. *How will this affect the family? How will we pay the mortgage? Where are we going to live? Who will look after the children? Will I be able to stand the pain?*

The situation can also be aggravated by less than optimal treatment by overworked and stressed hospital staff. It would be a very unusual cancer patient – or patient with any life-threatening disease – who was not stressed.

The feelings of stress are often accompanied by the release of noradrenaline and cortisol, better known as the 'fight or flight hormones.' Unfortunately, in circular fashion, these hormones can also be fertilisers for cancerous tumours![2,4] So, stress is not only suppressing the immune system, but it is also creating an environment that encourages the growth of the tumours. Stress reduction is therefore a priority, particularly when facing cancer.

Supplemental care
An important tool in the management of stress is the use of plant sterols and antioxidants found in Immuno-Care®.

Beta-sitosterol and stress-related disorders:
Research studies show that beta-sitosterol reduces the excessive release of cortisol, thus decreasing blood levels of cortisol.[5] Research also shows that:

* Phytonutrients raise DHEA levels and lower the cortisol: DHEA ratio, which indicates a more adaptive response to stress. [6]

- Beta-sitosterol protects against excessive inflammatory response found in high performance, physically-stressed athletes. [6]
- Beta-sitosterol protects the immune system against the stress response by stimulating the activity and proliferation of CD4 T-cells and NK cells to combat infection. [7]
- Beta-sitosterol can decrease the absorption of cholesterol in the digestive system and decrease the amount of cholesterol produced by the liver as a stress response. [8,9]
- Beta-sitosterol inhibits atherosclerosis.[10]

If you are diagnosed with a serious illness, take charge so that you do not feel so helpless. Find a good friend and a support group so that you do not feel so lonely.

Learn how to manage stress

You may feel like the stress in your life is out of your control, but there is something you can control: how you respond to it. Managing stress is all about taking charge: taking charge of your thoughts, your emotions, your schedule, your environment, and the way you deal with problems. Stress management involves changing the stressful situation when you can, changing your reaction when you can't, taking care of yourself, and making time for rest and relaxation.

Fortunately, since I (Alan) travelled this road, the problems arising from stress have been recognised and there have been some interesting studies addressing this issue. One particularly interesting one showed that slowing respiration to six cycles per minute synchronises inherent cardiovascular rhythms – meaning, slow down your breathing![10] It is not as difficult as you might imagine. Sit upright in a comfortable chair, feet flat on the floor.

Try to physically relax your feet, legs, shoulders (especially the shoulders!), neck and face. Then, inhale to the count of four. Pause. Then, "out, two, three, four." Pause again. Slow your breathing to a rate of approximately ten seconds a cycle.

At the same time, imagine a pleasant scene – whatever soothes you: a garden in summer, a lake surrounded by mountains, someone you love standing just behind you, or a favourite piece of music. You will be surprised how your heart rate will slow, and the stress will drain down out of your feet. Initially, try to do it for just a few minutes each day, then extend the time to ten to fifteen minutes morning and evening daily.

Many cancer centres now run Mindfulness-Based Stress Reduction (MBSR) programs , which can be a tremendous help, not only in reducing stress, but also to assure you that you are not alone on this journey.

Support groups also allow you to discuss the merits of complementary therapies, and be warned of the occasional charlatan who preys on vulnerable cancer patients and their loved ones. It is vital, however, that the group is a 'positive' group: a group where participants can confidentially express their concerns, provide emotional support and exchange some jokes. Laughter is a great medicine.

For the caregiver

When cancer has been diagnosed, it can be a particularly lonely time for the patient's partner. In a way, the patient has to do the work, take the treatments and do the healing, while the other partner is on the sidelines, worried sick. It can be very helpful to read some books together, a chapter at a time, and then discuss the chapter. This way the partners can travel the journey together, and it is no longer such a lonely journey for either partner. Books to consider reading include: Bernie Siegel's *Peace, Love, and Healing*, Alan Hobson's *Climb Back from Cancer*, and David Servan-Schreiber's *Anti-Cancer, A New Way of Life.*

It can also be very helpful to have a good friend who does not live with you, who you can 'dump on' from time to time, and who can sympathise with you. Or perhaps your friend will tell you to 'smarten up' – and then go home without worrying about the consequences!

So first thing, a battle plan: you take charge so that you do not feel so helpless. Find a good friend and a support group so that you do not feel so lonely.

Be grateful for your body

When you think about it, the body is a really remarkable creation. It can automatically balance as you walk, run or jump. Think of skaters doing spins and jumps, or the co-ordination of tennis players. Or a symphony orchestra with all those people playing exactly the right notes, (and there are many to choose from) all in exactly the right place, and all at exactly the right time – amazing. By detecting and differentiating tiny differences in high frequency vibrations in the air, your body enables you to hear. By detecting and differentiating very high frequencies of electromagnetic vibration, your body enables you to see. It truly is a miracle on two feet, and hey – you've been given this miracle as a gift!

Somebody once said to me that "inspiration is a blinding flash of the obvious!" Remember that your body really is amazing, and it is your best friend. So give it a hug, and say, "Thank you for being there for me."

---

[1] Palacios R, Sugarwara I. Hydrocortisone Abrogates Proliferation of T Cells in Autologous Mixed Lymphocyte Reaction by Rendering the Interleukin-2 Producer T Cells Unresponsive to Interleukin-1 and Unable to Synthesize the T-Cell Growth Factor. *Scanda. Jnl. Immunology*. 2006 Jun 1365-3083.

[2] Glasser R. Stress-associated Immune Dysregulation. *Brain Behav. Imm*. 2005 19;(1): 3-11.

[3] Marucha PT, Kiecolt-Glaser JK et al. Mucosal Wound Healing is Impaired by Examination Stress. *Psychosom. Med*. 1998 May-Jun 60;(3):62-5.

[4] Calcagni E, Elenkov I. Stress System Activity, Innate and T-Helper Cytokines, and Susceptibility to Immune Related Diseases. *Ann NY Acad. Sci*. 2006 Jun; 1069:62-76.

[5] Bouic PJD, Clark A, Lamprecht J, Freestone M et al. The effects of ß-sitosterol (BSS) and ß-sitosterol glucoside (BSSG) mixture on selected immune parameters of marathon runners: inhibition of post marathon immune suppression and inflammation. *Int J Sports Med*. 1999 (20):258-62.

[6] Gupta MB et al. Anti-inflammatory and anti-pyretic activities of ß-sitosterol. *Planta Med*. 1980 (39):157-163.

[7] Bouic PJD, Etsebeth S, Liebenberg RW et al. Beta-sitosterol and Beta-sitosterol glycoside stimulate human peripheral blood lymphocyte proliferation: implications for their use as an immunomodulatory vitamin combination. *Int J Immunopharmacol*. 1996 (18):693-700.

[8] Mattson FH et al. Optimizing the Effect of Plant Sterols on Cholesterol Absorption in Man. *Am J Clin Nutr*. 1982 (35):697-700.

[9] Murphy EA et al. The effects of sitosterol on serum cholesterol, platelet economy, thrombogenesis and atherosclerosis in the rabbit. *Atherosclerosis*. 1973 Mar-Apr (17);2: 257-268.

[10] Bernardi L, Sleight P et al. Effect of rosary prayer and yoga mantras on autonomic cardiovascular rhythms: comparative study. *BMJ* . 2001 Dec 22; 323(7327): 1446–1449.

[11] Besedovsky H, del Ray A. Physiology of psychoneuroimmunology: A personal view. *Brain Behav Imm* 2007 (21):34-44.

[12] Padgett DA, Glasser R. How stress influences the immune response. *Trends Immunol*. 2003 Aug; 24(8):444-8.

[13] Yang EV, Glasser R. Stress-induced immunomodulation: Implications for tumorigenesis. Brain Behav Immun. 2003 Feb;17 Suppl 1S37-S40.

[14] Antoni MH, Lutgendorf SK, Cole SW et al. The influence of bio-behavioural factors on tumour biology. *Nat Rev Cancer*. 2006 Mar 6(3): 240-8.

[15] Reiche EM, Morimoto HK, Nunes SM. Stress and depression-induced immune dysfunction: implications for the development and progression of cancer. *Int Rev Psychiatry*. 2005 Dec;17(6):515-27.

[16] Moreno-Smith M, Lutgendorf K, Sood AK. Impact of stress on cancer metastasis. *Future Oncol*. 2010, Dec;6(12): 1863

[17] Armaiz-Pena GN, Lutgendorf S, *et al.* Neuroendocrine modulation of cancer progression. *Brain Behav Immun.* 2009 Jan;23(1):10-15.

[18] Thaker PH, Sood AK. Neuroendocrine influences on cancer biology. *Semin Cancer Biol* 2008 Jun; 18(3) :164-70.

CHAPTER **FOUR**
🍃 **What's in Immuno-Care®?**

So far, we've explained what your immune system is, and what it requires in order to achieve peak performance. Unfortunately, because of the constant exposure to toxic chemicals, electropollution, processed food and other stressors, your immune system likely isn't getting all the nutrients it needs to keep you as healthy as possible. That's where Immuno-Care® comes in. This patented blend of nutrients works synergistically to support immune system health.

Plant Sterols

As mentioned previously, plant sterols are one of the most amazing health discoveries from the plant kingdom. Clinical studies have shown that patients deficient in phytonutrients rapidly become depleted of beta-sitosterol.[1]

This implies that these nutrients should be taken daily. An insufficient dietary intake could decrease the amount of plant sterols in the body with a consequent deterioration of health.

Now, plant sterols have been found to be an amazing helper in treating various modern diseases, as these natural organic compounds can modulate the body's immune system. Sterols (particularly beta-sitosterol) are one of the active ingredients in Immuno-Care®.

Beta-sitosterol, the principal phytosterol in most higher plants and hence in plant-derived food products, is found in the serum and tissues of healthy humans. Only plants can synthesize these compounds: humans and animals must obtain them from their diet. "Their apparent synergistic stimulatory effect on the immune system and prophylactic effect on a variety of diseases of civilisation indicates their importance in human and animal nutrition," says Dr. John Wilkinson, Senior Herbal Medicine Lecturer at Middlesex University, London, England.

"Since modern food processing tends to reduce their concentration in processed plant-food products, and eating habits also affect their consumption products adversely, it is desirable to eat sufficient unrefined or unprocessed plant foods, or resort to food supplements containing sitosterol. A good quality diet providing mainly unprocessed plant foods should readily supply a daily amount of 200-300mg plant sterols." [2]

> Plant sterols are a very exciting discovery. Worldwide research over the past 20 years has found that plant sterols strengthen the body's immune system, without any toxicity or side effects.
>
> *Dr. John Wilkinson,*
> *Middlesex University*

Here comes the sun

A topic that is not much discussed these days, but is important to human health, is the depletion of the ozone layer and the consequent increased intensity of the radiation coming from the sun. The United

Nations Environment Program's (UNEP) report on *The Effects of Increased Solar Ultraviolet Radiation on Human Health* opens with the statement: "The increase in UV-B associated with stratospheric ozone depletion is likely to have a substantial impact on human health." [3]

The report describes animal experiments in which UV exposure decreases the immune response to skin cancers, infectious agents, and other antigens. Likewise, suppressed immunity may occur either locally in sun-exposed skin or systematically at non-exposed sites, suggesting a link to increased skin cancer rates. [4]

So we have the situation in developed countries where, in the last few decades, the human diet has changed from mainly a *plant*-based diet to mainly a *processed food*-based diet that is low on these essential micronutrients; at the same time, the human body's immune system is under increasing attack, not only from herbicides, pesticides and other chemical irritants, but also from increased radiation. This may be the reason we have seen such a major increase in the incidence of autoimmune diseases over the last few years.

The UNEP report further states: "The growing evidence that the balance of Th-1 and Th-2 type immune responses plays an important role in determining the outcome of various infectious diseases, and that UV radiation may shift this balance towards a Th-2 type response suggests that UV radiation may indeed influence the pathogenesis of some diseases. It may also influence the outcome of vaccinations against infections."

In simple language, too much UV exposure impacts the immune system in a negative way. Here is why:

T-cells are part of the immune system; they recognize foreign bacteria and they produce cytokines (hormonal messengers) that are responsible for biological effects in the immune system. The cytokines fall into two groups: those that are pro-inflammatory, and those that are anti-inflammatory. In a well-functioning immune system, Th-1 and Th-2 cytokines are both produced by the helper T-cells, and work together to keep everything in balance.

What Do the Th-1 Cytokines Do?

The Th-1 type cells produce inflammation to kill viruses and certain bacteria, such as *Listeria* and *Mycobacterium tuberculosis* – the *bacillus* that causes tuberculosis. These cells also perpetuate any form of autoimmune response, and can cause cell-mediated allergies.

What Do the Th-2 Cytokines Do?

The Th-2 cytokines counteract the effects of the Th-1 cytokines, providing an anti-inflammatory action. But they also help kill extracellular pathogens, which live outside the body's cells and are exposed to antibodies in blood and other body fluids.

The Th-2 cytokines induce a pronounced allergic response. If you suffer from IgE-mediated allergies, or asthma, you are likely to be over-producing Th-2 types of cytokines, and have a Th-2 weighted imbalance. As an example, Th-2 cell predominance is found in people with systemic lupus erythematosus and allergic diseases.

Wired up

A more serious radiation threat than solar radiation is the 'home-grown' radiation arising particularly from cell phones, but also from TV transmissions, microwaves, etc. Your cell phone only receives your calls, but your body receives everyone's calls. The same is true of your TV: it only displays one station at a time, but your body is receiving the transmissions from many more stations.

This radiation causes ionization in the body, which in turn causes free radicals and the associated oxidative stress that gives rise to the pro-inflammatory cytokine interleukin-6 (IL-6). These free radicals can also be perceived as toxins by the body, giving rise to a further Th-2 response.

Researchers Breytenbach and Clark have shown that plant sterols can compensate for this shift in immune response due to solar radiation. Plant sterols have the potential to rebalance the immune system and shift a predominately Th-2 response to a predominately Th-1 response. [5]

Plant sterols, and in particular beta-sitosterol, have also been associated with a reduction of the pro-inflammatory cytokine IL-6, which is produced by oxidative stress.[6] (See also *University of Guelph Study*, Appendix 1). Research has shown phytonutrients to have important immunomodulatory, anti-inflammatory, anti-ulcer, anti-diabetic and anti-cancer properties. They are thought to be responsible for the health benefits of a variety of medicinal herbs including saw palmetto, pygeum, pumpkin seeds, devil's claw, milk thistle, ginkgo, panax and *Siberian ginseng*.

Understanding antioxidants

All antioxidants are not alike. Single source, alcohol-extracted antioxidants are derived from either single source plants or single source chemistry and are alcohol or solvent extract derivatives. Alcohol/solvent extract technology results in extracts that have mainly large molecular structures and are chemically singular in nature, and therefore, have a very narrow focus. Most alcohol extracts either function as an antioxidant or as a cellular cleanser. Very few (if any at all) have the ability to do both.

With single source, alcohol-extracted antioxidants, one out of ten people will have a very good response, two out of ten will have an average response, one out of ten will have some minimum response, and six out of ten will have no response at all. In addition, some solvents used for plant extract technology can be toxic to both humans and the environment.

Enzogenol™ - The Wide Spectrum Antioxidant

Enzogenol™ is a unique antioxidant supplement. The University of Canterbury's patented process creates an aqueous extract from *Pinus radiata* (pine bark), a superior source of proanthocyanidins and flavonoids.[7] Proanthocyanidins are plant nutrients that help to protect the plant from the perils of animal and biological predators. They have potent antioxidant and immune-boosting properties, and increase the activity of endogenous (internal) antioxidants such as glutathione and superoxide dismutase (SOD). Glutathione is important for cleaning and protecting cells from the inside, even immune cells themselves. SOD protects cells from free radical damage.

Flavonoids are the pigments that give plants their colour, and research shows they provide plenty of health benefits. For example, the flavonoid quercetin is helpful in stabilizing the cells that release histamine, providing an anti-inflammatory effect. The advanced antioxidant technology used to create Enzogenol™ provides free radical scavengers that are superior to other antioxidant technologies.

Flavonoids may play a beneficial role in the prevention or treatment of:

- allergies
- asthma
- atopic dermatitis
- cataracts
- diabetes
- gout
- macular degeneration
- migraine
- periodontal disease
- stomach ulcer

Enzogenol™ contains more of the higher molecular weight proanthocyanidins than any other antioxidant supplement. Enzogenol™ contains more than 90% of all known polyphenols, which are essential to proper human nutrition and may play a role in preventing degenerative conditions by enhancing the immune system. Recent studies provide evidence that increased consumption of polyphenols can reduce the risk of prostate, breast, lung and digestive cancers. [8, 9]

Benefits of the Pure Water Extraction Process

Aqueous extracts contain water-soluble 'small molecule' organic acids and compounds that are not found in solvent extracts. The body's uptake of phytonutrients derived from aqueous extract technology is significantly higher due to the soluble source (water), which the body's digestive system recognizes and transfers to cellular activity.

The small molecular-sized 'polyphenolic' molecules that are extracted by means of the new aqueous technology are normally more bioavailable and are much more potent and health promoting than extracts from alcohol or other solvent sources.[10]

Benefits of Enzogenol™

In addition to scavenging free radicals, Enzogenol™ can stimulate phagocytosis, an immune system response in which cells ingest and eliminate harmful micro-organisms and foreign heavy metals. It also has a powerful cleansing action that is known to be beneficial to the liver. The liver is the most important organ in the body for assimilation and distribution of antioxidants and cleansers to the cells. As its main function is to decrease toxins in the blood stream, however, it is very important that the liver be kept in good condition.

Research has also shown the amazing ability of this aqueous extract to inhibit the oxidation of low lipoproteins, the so-called 'bad' cholesterol involved in arterial heart disease.

Enzogenol™ has a unique phytochemical composition that is very specific to this particular species of *Pinus radiata*. Low molecular-sized molecules found in this specific extract are very effective against N-nitroso compounds (nitrosamines) that are found mainly in preserved meats like hot dogs, bacon, sausages, prepared sandwich meats and any smoked or barbequed foods, as well as many processed foods. Nitrosamines are known carcinogens. Enzogenol™ is also a very effective scavenger of free radicals activated by tobacco smoke and other lung-ingested carcinogens.

Antioxidants and your immune system

Antioxidants maintain the integrity and function of membrane lipids, cellular proteins, and nucleic acids. They also maintain control of signal transduction of gene expression in immune cells. For this reason, the immune cells are particularly sensitive to changes in their antioxidant status. Since the immune cells have a high percentage of polyunsaturated fatty acids in their plasma membrane, it is not surprising that these cells usually contain higher concentrations of antioxidants than do other cells.[11]

Thus, antioxidants play a vital role in maintaining immune cells in a reduced environment and protecting them from oxidative stress.

Enzogenol™ is a unique antioxidant complex because:

1. It is a wide-spectrum antioxidant, providing the largest range of flavonoids yet discovered (the most potent being the polyphenolic flavonoids).
2. It is derived through a pure water extraction process rather than a solvent-based process.
3. It has the capacity to stimulate phagocytosis and to cleanse the liver.
4. It is an effective scavenger of free radicals activated by ingested carcinogens.

Recent clinical trials have found that antioxidant supplementation can significantly improve certain immune responses.[12,13] Likewise, flavonoids, a major group of the antioxidants in Immuno-Care®, can also support the vascular system, as oxygen radicals can oxidise LDL, which injures the endothelial wall and thereby promotes atherosclerotic changes.[14]

Cellasate™
Just Passing Through?

Here's the problem.

After a supplement is swallowed, it is processed by the stomach acids. Plant sterols in their natural state are bound within the fibres of plants and fruits, and protected from destruction by the stomach acids. In supplements, they are no longer protected and are frequently destroyed.

(As an aside, all antioxidants are not the same. For instance, ascorbic acid, better known as Vitamin C, is an antioxidant that in a supplement would react with plant sterols to form sterol esters, which are only effective for a limited time. [15] However, Enzogenol™ has two main advantages: it consists of mainly proanthocyanidin complexes that are synergistic with plant sterols, and it is manufactured through an aqueous extraction process that leaves no residues).

The supplement then proceeds through to the small intestine where it is absorbed by the digestive system and enters the hepatic portal system. It is then carried through the portal vein into the liver before it reaches the rest of the body. The liver metabolizes the supplement, sometimes to such an extent that only a small amount of active ingredient emerges from the liver to the rest of the circulatory system. This *first pass* through the liver can greatly reduce the bioavailability of a supplement.

You are *not* what you eat: you are what you absorb.	More isn't always better, and less isn't often enough! What is important is *absorption*! Often, only small amounts of supplements

are actually absorbed by the body, and – you guessed it – the remainder goes down the toilet!

Factors inhibiting absorption

Mal-absorption in the gastrointestinal system can be caused by any or a combination of the following factors:

- High fat diet of processed and fast foods
- Lack of essential fibre in the diet
- Prescription drugs that cause depletion of friendly flora and enzymes in the digestive tract
- High stress factors
- Lack of proper exercise
- Chemical intervention from air and water pollution
- Surgery, radiation or chemotherapy.

The antioxidants incorporated into Immuno-Care® contain hydroxyl groups that can easily be destroyed by stomach acids. So, the first problem is how to protect the sterols. This is where we can take a leaf from the pharmaceutical industry that solved this problem a long time ago with *enteric coating*. Enteric coating provides a protective layer on a tablet as it passes through the stomach. Once the tablet reaches the duodenum (small intestine), the coating reacts to the alkaline environment and strips away, harmlessly releasing the contents of the tablet.

Some experts believe that due to damage from stomach acid, only 10 to 15% of the active ingredients in a pill or tablet actually get into the bloodstream. So why is enteric coating rarely used with nutritional supplements? Cost and knowledge! It's a very expensive technology and since most supplements are made to a price point that appeals to the general public (there is no medical insurance coverage for supplements), many manufacturers choose not to use it.

There are four effective ways in which nutrients can get into your bloodstream:
- via injection
- via the mucous membranes of the mouth
- via the lining of the walls of the colon (suppositories)
- via the lining of the walls of the upper intestine.

High quality supplements are formulated to allow much higher levels of bioavailability than cheaper, mass-produced vitamin and mineral products. This is because they are science-based and use more sophisticated manufacturing processes. This is one reason why they cost more – but work better! Reputable supplement companies, however, always manufacture in line with GMP (good manufacturing practices) and pharmaceutical standards. It's important to check on this when evaluating and comparing supplements!

The kilogram capsule?

To obtain a therapeutic response to certain compounds, dosage range is critical. Some manufacturers of plant sterols will tell you that a 20mg capsule taken three times per day is an appropriate dosage, while others will tell you that a 450mg capsule twice per day is an ideal dosage. So how far will some of the manufacturers go with sterol dosages? Are we close to the big kilogram capsule? I'm sure most of us would not look forward to taking a kilogram capsule three or four times a day! Fortunately, research shows that 300mg of plant sterols is the optimum daily intake.[2]

Enteric coating and the inclusion of Cellasate™, designed to facilitate the absorption and retention of the sterols and antioxidants in Immuno-Care®, ensures that the body actually absorbs these ingredients. The peptides contained within Cellasate™ have an extremely strong influence in balancing the immune system, especially in people with allergies and auto-immune disorders. The improved balance of the gastrointestinal system and the additional support for the immune system, come as a bonus.

[1] Salen G, Ahrens EH, Grundy SM. Metabolism of beta-sitosterol in man. *J Clin Invest*. 1970 May; 49(5):952-967.

[2] Pegel KH. The importance of sitosterol and sitosterolin in human and animal nutrition. *SA J Sci*. 1997(93):263-268.

[3] Longstreth JD et al. Human health. Chapter 2 in *Environmental effects of ozone depletion: 1991 update*, 15-24. United Nations Environment Programme (UNEP).

[4] Kripke ML, Morison WL. Modulation of the immune function by UV radiation. *J Invest Dermatol*. 1985 Jul; 85 (1 Suppl):62s-66s.

[5] Breytenbach U, Clark A et al. Flow Cytometric Analysis of the Th-1/Th-2 Balance in Healthy Individuals. *Cell Biol Interntl*. 2001; 25(1):43-49.

[6] Devaraj S, Autret BC, Jialal I. Reduced-calorie orange juice beverage with plant sterols lowers C-reactive protein concentrations and improves the lipid profile in human volunteers. *Am J Clin Nutr*. 2006 Oct;84(4):756-61.

[7] Enzogenol™. A natural extract of *Pinus radiata* pine bark - an overview. Enzo Nutraceuticals Ltd. www.enzogenol.com

[8] Markham KR, Porter LJ. Extractives of *Pinus radiata* bark. I. Phenolic components. *NZ J Sci*. 1973 Dec;16(4):751-761.

[9] Porter LJ. Extractives of *Pinus radiata* bark. Proanthocyanadin constituents. *NZ J Sci*. 1974 (70):213-218.

[10] Williams VM, Porter LJ, Hemingway RW. Molecular weight profiles of proanthocyanadin polymers. *Phytochem* 1983;22(2):569-572.

[11] De La Fuente M, Victor VM. Antioxidants as modulators of immune function. *Immunol Cell Biol* 2000 Feb;78:49-54.

[12] Bendrich, A. Beta-carotene and the immune response. *Proc Nutr Soc*. 1991 (50)2:263-274.

[13] Nijveldt RJ et al. Flavonoids: a review of probable mechanisms of action and potential applications. *Am J Clin Nutr*. 2001 Oct;74(4):418-425.

[14] Loscalzo J. Oxidant stress: a key determinant of artherothrombosis. *Biochem Soc Trans*. 2003 Oct; 31(pt 5):1059-61.

[15] O'Neill FH et al. Comparison of the effects of dietary plant sterol and stanol esters on lipid metabolism. *Nutr Metab Cardiovasc Dis*. 2004 Jun;14(3):133-142.

PART TWO: Research

CHAPTER **FIVE**

Allergies and Asthma

A staggering number of people around the world suffer from allergies. In North America alone, there are approximately 30 million allergy sufferers, and the figure is growing. No one is born with an allergy, but you can have a genetic tendency to develop one. If both your parents have allergies, you will have a 75% chance of also developing them.

Allergies explained

There are two types of allergic response: the first is a classic allergic response in which the allergen triggers an increase in immunoglobulin E (IgE), and the reaction is immediate. Allergens can initiate different symptoms depending on where they settle in the body. An upper respiratory tract irritation will trigger sneezing and a runny nose, while the same allergen in the lower respiratory tract will produce wheezing or coughing.

The second type of allergic response is cell-mediated or delayed-onset response. This is more difficult to diagnose, as the symptoms may not occur immediately. These symptoms tend to be in the gastrointestinal tract in the form of gastric upsets, diarrhea, irritable bowel, etc.

Allergies are nothing to sneeze about

Allergies are rarely life-threatening, but serious allergic reactions can occur. These include swelling of the respiratory passages, shortness of breath, and anaphylactic reaction. People who suffer from allergies have an increased chance of developing respiratory infections and may be more susceptible to developing asthma. The majority of allergy sufferers are affected by reduced efficiency in daily activities, decreased energy levels, and a reduced quality of life.

Common allergens

Common allergens in the air are pollen, mould, animal dander and dust. Many other things can make your allergy symptoms worse. Pollen comes from trees, grass and weeds. Allergies that occur in the spring (late April and May) are often due to tree pollen. Allergies that occur in the summer (late May to mid-July) are often due to grass and weed pollen. Allergies that occur in the fall (late August to the first frost) are often due to weed pollen.

Mould is common where water tends to collect, such as shower curtains, window moldings and damp basements. It can also be found on rotting logs, hay, mulches, commercial peat moss, compost piles and leaf litter. An allergy to mould is usually worse during humid and rainy weather. West coast USA and Canada and the Atlantic areas usually experience allergic reactions to winter moulds.

Another common allergen, animal dander, is made up of bits of skin and hair from pets. You can be exposed to dander when handling an animal or from house dust that contains dander.

Dust contains allergens, including dust mites. Dust mites are tiny living creatures found in bedding, mattresses, carpets and furniture. They like places where it's warm and humid. They live on dead skin cells and other things found in house dust. Aerosol sprays, perfumes, air pollution, cold air, humidity, fumes, tobacco smoke, wind and wood smoke can make allergies feel worse.

Meet the cast
Interleukin-6

The immune system responds to stressors by causing certain immune cells to secrete the pro-inflammatory cytokines, Interleukin-1 (IL-1) and Interleukin-6 (IL-6). These cytokines are both involved in inflammation and IL-6 is thought to worsen symptoms of autoimmune diseases and fibromyalgia.[1,2]

Interleukin-6 has been found to act as a growth factor in several tumours, and some viruses use IL-6 to replicate. IL-6 also causes calcium to be released from bone, thus promoting osteoporosis. Control of the release of these cytokines is necessary to enhance immunity and reduce degenerative diseases.

Basophils

Basophils are a type of white blood cell produced in the bone marrow. Basophils help to protect the body from bacteria and parasites, but they can cause problems when they react against harmless substances, leading to allergies, asthma, and other inflammatory reactions in the body.

"Merci infiniment" for sending me your exceptional product, Immuno-Care®. On the third day, my symptoms were reduced by at least 80%. Today, my energy has returned and I don't have any pain anymore in my back: no sneezing, no watery eyes or running nose and no headache. I feel myself again.

S., Montreal, QC

Basophils release histamine, which increases the permeability of the capillaries to white blood cells. This increased permeability causes fluid to escape into tissues, leading to the classic runny nose and watery eyes associated with an allergic reaction. Not meant to annoy you, this reaction is designed to flush potential threats out of your body.

Along with releasing histamine, basophils secrete lipid mediators like leukotrienes, and several cytokines. Each of these substances contributes to inflammation.

I have suffered with allergies for years. I have only been taking your supplement for 5 days and cannot explain the difference that I feel. Can you tell me what is in this supplement that makes my allergy symptoms almost non-existent? I have had the flu and a cold for the past 6 months and could not get my feet on the ground when I came across your product. Insomnia was another issue which I think this is helping with.

T.M., Ontario

Recent evidence suggests that basophils are an important source of the cytokine, Interleukin-4, perhaps more important than T-cells. Basophils are responsible for the development of IgE – mediated chronic allergic inflammation independently of T-cells and mast cells. Interleukin-4 is considered one of the critical cytokines in the development of allergies and the production of IgE antibody by the immune system.

Basophils readily generate large quantities of TH-2 cytokines, providing new insights into the possible role of basophils in allergic diseases and immunity to pathogens.[3,4,5]

Mast cells
The mast cell is the cornerstone of

allergic disease, particularly near surfaces exposed to the environment (mucous membranes, nose, mouth, skin). Along with basophils, mast cells are found in connective tissue and are a type of white blood cell. It's thought that both mast cells and basophils originate from bone marrow. Basophils leave the bone marrow already mature, whereas the mast cell circulates in an immature form, only maturing once in a tissue site. The site at which an immature mast cell settles probably determines the precise characteristics of the mast cell.

In response to an allergen, coarse granules within mast cells release histamine (as well as serotonin, bradykinin and heparin). Of these, histamine is the most familiar to allergy sufferers. Its role is to widen blood capillaries and increase their permeability so fluids can pass from the blood to the tissues, causing swelling. Histamine is also responsible for the involuntary contraction of smooth muscles, for example, in the lungs. Histamine poses challenges in allergies because it's reacting to what is otherwise a harmless substance.

Asthma

Asthma and allergies are related, but they are not the same thing. An allergy is a reaction to a substance that

A 60-year-old woman consulted my office with a shoulder problem and terrible allergies. Clinically, this area can be associated with sinus problems. I did a chiropractic adjustment and follow up, with no changes to her allergies. I then suggested she try Immuno-Care® as part of the treatment plan. After 1 week of taking 4 capsules per day, she reported a 90% improvement in her symptoms. Bottom line: the patient is thrilled.

Dr R.A., Kelowna BC

is usually harmless. These substances (allergens) can be inhaled, injected, swallowed, or touched. Being exposed to an allergen may cause irritation and swelling in specific areas of the body, such as the nose, eyes, lungs, and skin. Allergens like pollen, mould, animal dander and dust mites can make asthma symptoms worse by increasing the inflammation in the airways and making them more sensitive. The best way to find out if you are allergic to something is to have an allergy assessment done.

Many people with asthma also have allergies and your doctor may refer you to an allergist if you are experiencing asthma symptoms. However, just as not everyone who has allergies develops asthma, not everyone who has asthma has allergies. Researchers are still trying to determine the exact relationship between the two, but many people do suffer from both.

Each person's asthma triggers are different, and an important part of managing the condition is identifying what your triggers are. Some triggers are considered inflammatory, meaning they cause mucous and inflammation in the airways.[6,7,8,9]

> I have been on puffers and inhalers for many years, and although these things helped me, I never felt they worked as well as they should and so I suffered with severe asthma symptoms. I work for a US distributor of natural medicines, and after realizing that this product may help me with asthma, I decided to give it a try. It only took 2 weeks for my symptoms to subside noticeably. After a few months of use, I was breathing easier; I could exercise more and in general felt I was finally getting control of my symptoms. I would highly recommend this product.
>
> *Scott Saunders, Mill Creek, Washington, USA*

Abstract from Guelph Trial

A randomized double-blind, placebo-controlled clinical trial on Immuno-Care® was completed at the University of Guelph, Ontario, Canada.

This pilot study was conducted at the Human Nutraceutical Research Unit and was designed to investigate the effect of supplementation with Immuno-Care® on immunological response to allergens. There were 20 participants in the study. When compared to the control group, participants in the treatment group showed a statistically significant reduction in the basophils that are responsible for histamine release.

The recommended dose during the trial was a loading dose of one capsule in the morning, and one capsule in the evening for 7 consecutive days. Participants were then advised by the research team to reduce the dosage to one capsule per day for the duration of the study.

The research also showed a substantial reduction in the pro-inflammatory cytokine IL-6 levels in the treatment group when compared to the control group:

Immune Parameters	Immuno-Care® Day 0	Immuno-Care® Day 28	Immuno-Care® Difference Day 28-Day 0	Control Day 0	Control Day 28	Control % Difference Day 28-Day 0
IL-6	1.261	0.937	-25.7%	1.318	1.179	10.5%
Eosinophils	0.24	0.20	-16.7%	0.23	0.20	-13.0%
Basophils	0.23	0.01	- 95.6%**	0.13	0.04	- 69%

** statistically significant, $p < 0.05$

Immuno-Care® has demonstrated that it has an effect on histamine release from human basophils and also on IL-6 levels, and consequently can substantially alleviate symptoms associated with airborne allergens. Further studies will be conducted with a larger patient population and a longer trial period to investigate other areas of immunological response.

Phytonutrients taken in their proper dosage of 300mg per day have been shown to be very effective in preventing allergies. Enzogenol™, an ingredient in this product, is a powerful antioxidant that also helps in the control of allergies. Phytonutrients are proving to be very effective in halting allergies in a safe and natural way.[10]

Physicians who use this product claim that patient compliance using Immuno-Care® is excellent. That means people see results and stay on the product to really make sure they give it enough time to respond.

---

[1] Lin RY et al. Interleukin 6 and C-reactive protein levels in patients with acute allergic reactions: an emergency department-based study. *Ann Allergies Asthma Immunol.* 2001 Nov; 87(5):412-6.

[2] Wong CK et al. Proinflammatory cytokines and Th cytokines in patients with allergic asthma. *Clin Exp Immunol.* 2001 Aug;125(2):177-83.

[3] Mukai K et al. Basophils play a critical role in the development of IgE-mediated chronic allergic inflammation independently of T-cells and mast cells. *Immunity.* 2005 Aug;23(2):191-202.

[4] Obata K et al. Basophils are essential initiators of a novel type of chronic allergic inflammation. *Blood.* 2007Aug 1;110(3):913-20.

[5] Falcone FH et al. The 21st century renaissance of the basophil? Current insights into its role in allergic response and innate immunity. *Exp Dermatol.* 2006 Nov;15(11):855-64.

[6] Koshino T et al. Airway basophil and mast cell density in patients with bronchial asthma: relationship to bronchial hyperresponsiveness. *J Asthma* 1996; 33(2):89-95.

[7] Gauvreau GM et al. Increased numbers of both airway basophils and mast cells in sputum after allergen inhalation challenge of atopic asthmatics.. *Am J Respir Crit Care Med.* 2000 May;161(5):1473-8.

[8] Denburg JA. Basophils and mast cells in airway inflammation and asthma. *Can Respir J.* 1998 Jul-Aug; 5 Suppl A:41A-4A.

[9] Neveu WA et al. Elevation of IL-6 in the allergic asthmatic airway is independent of inflammation but associates with loss of central airway function. *Respir Res* 2010 Mar 8; 11:28.

[10] Kawai M et al. Flavonoids and related compounds as anti-allergic substances. *Allergol Int.* 2007 Jun;56(2):113-123.

CHAPTER **SIX**

Chronic Inflammation

Inflammation has classically been viewed as a short-term response to tissue injury that produces characteristic symptoms and usually resolves spontaneously. Interesting new research, however, shows chronic inflammation to be a major factor in the development of degenerative disease and loss of youthful functions. During the early days of researching Immuno-Care®, we became very interested in chronic inflammation and how inflammation itself is not a disease, but is featured to varying degrees, in adverse health conditions.

Of the ten leading causes of mortality in the United States in fact, chronic, low-level inflammation contributes to at least seven conditions, including heart disease, cancer, chronic lower respiratory disease, stroke, Alzheimer's disease, diabetes, and kidney disease. [1,2]

Before we get into a discussion of how chronic inflammation is health-damaging, let's first take a look at the purpose of the inflammatory process.

The acute inflammatory response

Inflammation is triggered by tissue injury (trauma, exposure to heat or chemicals) or infection by viruses, bacteria, parasites, or fungi.[3] The classic manifestation of acute inflammation is characterized by four principal signs:

1. Redness and heat result from the increased blood flow to the site of injury.
2. Swelling results from the accumulation of fluid at the injury site, a consequence of the increased blood flow.
3. Swelling can compress nerve endings near the injury, causing the characteristic pain associated with inflammation.
4. Pain is also important to make the organism aware of the tissue damage. Additionally, inflammation in a joint usually results in a fifth sign (impairment of function), which has the effect of limiting movement and forcing rest of the injured joint to aid in healing.

Inflammation has several protective functions as well as assisting in the repair process: it prevents the spread of infection and damage to nearby tissues, and helps to remove damaged tissue and pathogens.

When it becomes chronic

A third type of stimuli, known as cellular stress, triggers chronic inflammation which contributes to disease and age-related degeneration in a variety of ways. Cellular stress and dysfunction can be caused by excessive calorie consumption, elevated blood sugar levels, and oxidative stress. Research now suggests that a lower caloric diet may be a way to possibly reduce inflammatory reactions.[4]

Chronic inflammation is deceptive in that its silent nature conceals its destructive power. In fact, stress-induced inflammation, once triggered, can persist undetected for years or even decades, propagating cell death throughout the body. Due to the fact that it contributes so greatly to deterioration associated with the aging process, this silent state of chronic inflammation has been coined a 'silent killer.'

Cellular stress

Cell mitochondria are responsible for producing energy and mitochondrial dysfunction is a result of the aging process itself. Unfortunately, free radicals are a byproduct of mitochondrial energy generation. Free radicals can damage cellular structures and initiate a cascade of pro-inflammatory genetic signals that ultimately result in cell death or uncontrolled cell growth – the trademark of cancer.

Additional biochemical inducers of a chronic inflammatory response include:

- Homocysteine: a non-protein-forming amino acid that is a marker and risk factor for cardiovascular disease, and may increase bone fracture risk [5] (See *Heart Disease*)
- Uric acid (urate) crystals: can be deposited in joints during gouty arthritis; elevated levels are a risk factor for kidney disease, hypertension, and metabolic syndrome [6]
- Oxidized lipoproteins (such as LDL): a significant contributor to atherosclerotic plaques.[7] (See *Heart Disease*)

It is possible to reduce chronic inflammation and consequently reduce the risk for inflammatory diseases, by targeting some of the factors that can initiate the inflammatory responses. Some

I have had RA for some years and I have used the usual NSAIDS and other pain killers, but the results were minimal – and then I tried Immuno-Care®. I can honestly say the relief of pain is quite remarkable. Walking used to be my worst experience, as I have RA in the knees, hips, feet, hands and wrists. I am now able to walk without using any aids. I can resume needle work in moderation and even get in and out of buses/cars, and do some household chores. It is truly remarkable. One cannot adequately express pain relief. It is, in part, a feeling of having some joy back in life. The second best part of it all that there is no "adverse reactions" – it being a natural product and safe to use." *M.D., BC*

of these factors include interleukins and C-reactive protein. Interleukins are cytokines that have many functions in the promotion and resolution of inflammation. Interleukin-6 (IL-6) has both pro-inflammatory and anti-inflammatory roles, and coordinates the progression and resolution of acute inflammation. IL-6 is expressed by both immune and non-immune cells, and helps to attract neutrophils (immune cells that can destroy pathogens) to sites of injury.[8]

C-reactive protein (CRP), on the other hand, is an acute-phase protein, one of several proteins rapidly produced by the liver during an inflammatory response. Its primary goal in acute inflammation is to coat damaged cells so that they are more easily recognized by other immune cells.

CRP elevation above basal levels is not a diagnostic indicator on its own: it can be elevated in several cancers, rheumatologic, gastrointestinal, and cardiovascular conditions, and infections. Elevation of CRP has a strong association with elevated risk not only of cardiovascular disease, but also silent brain infarction, especially in the elderly. [9,10]

Risk factors for chronic inflammation

Age: In contrast to younger individuals (whose levels of inflammatory cytokines typically increase only in response to infection or injury), older adults can have consistently elevated levels of several inflammatory markers, especially IL-6 and TNF-α.[9] TNF-alpha is a member of a group of cytokines that stimulate inflammation, although the primary role of TNF-α is in the regulation of immune cells. The inflammatory response causes many of the clinical problems associated with autoimmune disorders such as rheumatoid arthritis, psoriasis, ankylosing spondylitis, inflammatory bowel disease (Crohn's disease), psoriatic arthritis and asthma.

These elevations are observed even in healthy older individuals. While the reasoning for this age-associated increase in inflammatory markers is not thoroughly understood, it may reflect cumulative mitochondrial dysfunction and oxidative damage, or may be the result of other risk factors associated with age, such as increases in body fat.

Obesity: Fat tissue can store and secrete multiple hormones and cytokines into circulation, affecting metabolism throughout the body. For example, fat cells produce

A study conducted at the University of Guelph showed that the pro-inflammatory cytokine Interleukin-6 was reduced in participants using Immuno-Care®, and therefore may contribute to a better feeling of wellness in people with chronic inflammatory conditions.

and secrete both TNF-α and IL-6. Visceral (abdominal) fat cells can produce three times the amount of IL-6 as fat cells elsewhere, and in overweight individuals, may be producing up to 35% of the total IL-6 in the body. [11]

Diet: A diet high in saturated fat is associated with higher pro-inflammatory markers, particularly in diabetic or overweight individuals.

In the Western world, dietary over-consumption is a major contributor to inflammation and other detrimental age-related processes. Eating a calorie-restricted diet without malnutrition, therefore, is an effective means of relieving physiologic stressors. Indeed, several studies show that calorie restriction provides powerful protection against inflammation. The current studies with rodents and some larger animals, as well as humans, now indicate you can probably extend your life expectancy potentially by up to 50% from eating a calorie-restricted diet.

When you restrict your calories, your body recognizes that it doesn't have resources to waste, and it gets more efficient. Cells also benefit when calories are limited: they don't have the same toxic waste products coming out of the energy cells, so individual cell lines live longer. This newly-discovered chemical pathway is called the *sirtuin pathway* – a family of enzymes that shows potential to extend lifespan while playing a key role in the body's natural defense against disease.

Consuming a limited number of calories (approximately 2,000 per day) while still getting enough of a range of specific nutrients, has been shown to extend the lives of creatures ranging from common fruit flies to rats to primates to humans.[12]

Smoking: Lighting up is an obvious health hazard that promotes inflammation, particularly reactive oxygen species. Smoking also increases the risk of periodontal disease, an independent risk factor for increasing systemic inflammation.

Sleep disorders: Production of inflammatory cytokines appears to follow a circadian rhythm and may be involved in the regulation of sleep. Disruption of normal sleep can lead to daytime elevations of these pro-inflammatory molecules.

Periodontal disease: Gum disease can produce a systemic inflammatory response that may affect several other systems, such as the heart and kidneys. It is by this mechanism that periodontal disease is a risk factor for cardiovascular diseases.[13]

Stress: Both physical and emotional stress can lead to inflammatory cytokine release (IL-6); stress is also associated with decreased sleep and increased body mass (stimulated by release of the stress hormone cortisol), both of which are independent causes of inflammation.[14,15]

Inflammation here and now

It would appear that many modern day diseases are associated with inflammation and it is important, therefore, to develop lifestyle choices that minimize the potential for inflammation to develop. Immuno-Care® can help.

---

[1] Centers for Disease Control and Prevention. FASTSTATS - Leading Causes of Death. *cdc.gov.* 2011. Available at: http://www.cdc.gov/NCHS/fastats

[2] Kundu JK, Surh YJ. Inflammation: gearing the journey to cancer. *Mutat Res.* 2008 Jul-Aug;659(1-2):15–30.

[3] Medzhitov R. Origin and physiological roles of inflammation. *Nature.* 2008;454(7203):428–435.

[4] Karin M, Lawrence T, Nizet V. Innate immunity gone awry: linking microbial infections to chronic inflammation and cancer. *Cell.* 2006 Feb 24;124(4):823–835.

[5] Au-Yeung KK et al. Folic acid inhibits homocysteine-induced superoxide anion production and nuclear factor kappa B activation in macrophages. *Can J Physiol Pharmacol.* 2006 Jan;84(1):141–147.

[6] Martinon F et al. Gout-associated uric acid crystals activate the NALP3 inflammasome. *Nature.* 2006;440(7081):237–241.

[7] Nguyen-Khoa T et al. Oxidized low-density lipoprotein induces macrophage respiratory burst via its protein moiety: A novel pathway in atherogenesis? *Biochem Biophys Res Commun.* 1999;263(3):804–809.

[8] Gabay C. Interleukin-6 and chronic inflammation. *Arthritis Res Ther.* 2006;8 Suppl 2:S3.

Harris TB, Ferrucci L et al. Associations of elevated interleukin-6 and C-reactive protein levels with mortality in the elderly. *Am J Med.* 1999 May;106(5):506-12.

[9] Hoshi T et al. Relations of Serum High-Sensitivity C-Reactive Protein and Interleukin-6 Levels With Silent Brain Infarction. *Stroke.* 2005; 36(4):768-772.

[10] Trayhurn, P et al. Signaling role of adipose tissue: adipokines and inflammation in obesity. *Biochem Soc Trans.* 2005;33(Pt 5):1078–1081.

[11] Mohamed-Ali, et al. Subcutaneous adipose tissue releases interleukin-6, but not tumor necrosis factor-alpha, in vivo. *J Clin Endocrinol Metab.* 1997;82(12):4196–4200.

[12] Giugliano, D et al. The Effects of Diet on Inflammation. *J Am Coll Cardiol.* 2006;48(4):677–685.

[13] Slade GD et al. Relationship between periodontal disease and C-reactive protein among adults in the Atherosclerosis Risk in Communities Study. *Arch Intern Med.* 2003;163(10):1172–1179.

[14] Pervanidou P, Chrousos GP et al. Metabolic consequences of stress during childhood and adolescence. *Metabolism.* 2011; Physiology of Psychoneuroimmunology.

[15] Padgett DA, Glaser R. How Stress Influences the Immune Response. *Trends in Imm.* 2003 Aug;24(8).

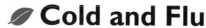 # Cold and Flu

Who wants to be a hermit? Not me!

It's true: the more people you come in contact with, the greater your chance of catching whatever is going around. At first, it might seem the only way to protect yourself from catching the cold or flu viruses each year is to become a hermit come winter. But have no fear, my friends. You can protect yourself from the annual cold and flu season.

The nasty bugs

There are some basic ways of minimizing your chances of catching these nasty viruses. Most times, we actually catch colds and flu by touching something with the virus on it. Does this mean we should go around paranoid of touching things like railings or washroom doors? Of course not! Washing your hands regularly is the simplest way to protect yourself, but, unfortunately, most people do not wash their hands regularly. Likewise, it's a good idea to avoid touching your eyes and nose, as this is generally how a virus is spread. You can also catch a virus through the air after someone sneezes, but there's not much you can do about that. Or is there?

Will you get a cold or flu this winter?

The odds are: yes, you will! North Americans will get an average of six colds per year. Although the typical life-cycle of a cold is a few days to two weeks, many of these colds and flu come from more difficult strains of a virus and seem to stay much longer in the body than they used to years ago. Alternatively, people can experience colds and flu that seem to have disappeared but return only a few weeks later. So are antibiotics the answer?

Drugs for cold and flu?

The *Journal of the American Medical Association* (*JAMA*) found that antibiotics have little or no benefit for colds and flu, or upper respiratory tract infections.[1] *JAMA* reported that the historical rate of antibiotic prescribing has even backfired, causing an increase of new, harmful, drug-resistant strains of bacteria.

In fact, a report in the prestigious British journal *The Lancet* mentioned two studies that raise significant concern regarding the flu. One says that the flu shot is really not that effective in the older population, which is the prime target population for vaccination. The other says that the drugs we have stockpiled in the event of a flu epidemic won't work now for many people because the flu viruses have become resistant to them.[2,3]

> **Did you know?**
> The connection between psychological stress and infection by respiratory viruses is clear. When the immune system is under stress, research shows that interleukin-6 is secreted by our immune system. Il-6 suppresses the immune function, allowing unwanted viruses to enter the body and cause illness.
> *Sheldon Cohen, MD*
> *Carnegie Mellon University*
> *of Pittsburgh*

According to the data presented in *The Lancet* in 2012, world-wide patient resistance to the medicines used to treat the flu have increased a whopping 12% in the past 10 years.

What to do?

Any doctor will tell you that the best defense against colds and flu and the fight against infection is to have a strong immune system. 'Curing' diseases with drugs often results in a reoccurrence of the same problem later, because the real cause of the disease was not addressed.

Even worse, because drugs can cause disease organisms to concentrate and mutate (creating resistant strains of pathogens), the disease or infection often recurs with a vengeance. Consequently, the most effective and safest way to be healthy is to strengthen the immune system using natural products so that you avoid catching colds or flu in the first place.

Just what the doctor ordered

Beta-sitosterol protects the immune system by stimulating the activity and proliferation of natural killer (NK) cells and CD-4 T-cells to combat infection.[1] CD-4 cells are white blood cells that signal other cells to destroy viruses. The formulation of phytonutrients, powerful natural antioxidants and a complex of essential fatty acids in Immuno-Care® are shown to be effective in the treatment of colds and flu. The symptoms associated with these conditions leave the body much quicker and the immune system goes into high gear to return the system to optimum health.

According to Dr Larry Bausch, San Diego, California, "This new product represents a quantum leap in nutraceutical technology. I am very thankful to be able to use it in my practice.

I have seen many natural remedies on the market that boost the immune system, but I have not seen one that is able to balance the immune system as well as Immuno-Care®. And while many products boost the immune system, that can be very harmful to people suffering from autoimmune diseases. I now prescribe Immuno-Care® to many of my patients, who are finding relief from immune system disorders. I also found that while my patients are being treated with Immuno-Care®, they are not catching colds and flu they once seemed to get."

I just wanted to tell you that your product probably saved my career! I teach (college level) and in the winter, with the sneezing and coughing and the closed windows and poor air circulation, I was catching five or six colds a year. I was basically sick all winter long. At one point in time, I was seriously considering retirement – even though I am only 47 years old and ages away from collecting a pension.

My sister suggested your product, which I started to take a few weeks before classes began in the fall. I have been cold-free for three consecutive winters now. Taking that little pill every morning has become an essential part of my routine. In fact, I don't think I would dare face another Canadian winter without it. I would have been forced to walk away from my teaching, the one thing that I truly like to do. God bless you for giving me that chance.

A.L., Montreal, QC

Supplement a healthy diet

Dr Bausch wonders, "How many of us eat the prescribed amount of fruit and vegetable recommended by Health Canada or the FDA? Not many! Some studies have shown that even vegetarians are not getting the right amount of phytonutrients. Our modern diets are also lacking in plant phytonutrients, as modern food processing destroys these vital health promoting nutrients." To promote optimal health, aim to eat 7-10 servings of fruits and vegetables daily.

"One important supplement that I recommend to my patients is Immuno-Care®," says Dr. Bausch. "I have worked with this product and I have seen this supplement work in my practice. Plant sterols at the proper dosage of 300mg, powerful antioxidants to fight free radical damage, and a complex of essential fatty acids to deliver the nutrients to the body's cell structure are what makes this a product that you should take on a daily basis."

---

[1] Gwaltney JM, Halstead SB. Contagiousness of the common cold. Invited letter in "Questions and Answers". *Journal of the American Medical Association* 278 (3): 256–257. 16 July 1997. http://jama.ama-assn.org/content/278/3/256

[2] Resistance to Anti-Flu Agents Increasing Worldwide, and Flu Vaccines Have Modest Effectiveness in Elderly People. *The Lancet*, Press Release September 20, 2005. www.thelancet.com

[3] Osterholm MT, Kelley NS, Sommer A, Belongia EA. Efficacy and effectiveness of influenza vaccines: a systematic review and meta-analysis. *Lancet Infect Dis.* 2012 Jan;12(1):36-44.

CHAPTER **EIGHT**

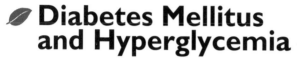

Diabetes Mellitus and Hyperglycemia

North America is in the midst of a diabetes epidemic. Over the past 20 years, the number of adults diagnosed with diabetes has more than doubled, and children are being diagnosed with diabetes in alarming numbers. Diabetes has rapidly emerged as a leading culprit in the epidemic of heart disease also sweeping the country.

It is crucial that diabetics (and those predisposed to diabetes) understand the ways in which blood glucose causes damage so you can take active steps to interrupt these processes.

Diabetes mellitus defined

Diabetes comes from Greek, and it means *siphon*. Aretus the Cappadocian, a Greek physician during the second century A.D., named the condition *diabainein*. He described patients who were passing too much water (polyuria) – like a siphon. The word became diabetes from the English adoption of the Medieval Latin *diabetes*.

In 1675, Thomas Willis added *mellitus* to the term, although today it is commonly referred to simply as diabetes. *Mel* in Latin means honey; the urine and blood of people with diabetes has excess glucose, and glucose is sweet like honey. *Diabetes mellitus* could litreally mean "siphoning off sweet water."

How diabetes happens

When our food is digested, the glucose makes its way into the bloodstream. Our cells use the glucose for energy and growth. However, glucose cannot enter our cells without insulin being present.

Insulin is a hormone produced by the pancreas. After eating, the pancreas automatically releases an adequate quantity of insulin to move the glucose in our blood into the cells, and lowers the blood sugar level.

A person with diabetes has a condition in which the quantity of glucose in the blood is too elevated (hyperglycemia). This is because the body does not produce enough insulin, produces no insulin, or has cells that do not respond properly to the insulin the pancreas produces. This results in too much glucose building up in the blood. This excess blood glucose eventually passes out of the body in urine. So, even though the blood has plenty of glucose, the cells are not getting it for their essential energy and growth requirements.

In ancient China, people observed that ants would be attracted to some people's urine, because it was sweet. The term 'sweet urine disease' was coined.

More to the story:
While hyperglycemia (high blood sugar) is considered the main cause of diabetes, another less well-known process called glycation is also a major factor in diabetes. Gly-

cation is a chemical reaction in which sugar-derived molecules react with proteins to produce advanced glycation end products (AGEs) or glycotoxins. The glycation process occurs very slowly in a normal healthy body, but for those suffering from diabetes, this process increases at a fast rate due to the fact that diabetics have abnormal glucose levels in their system. Glycation is a key feature of diabetes-related complications, and is linked to nerve damage, heart attack, and blindness. As an example, diabetics who smoke show significant AGEs deposits in their arteries and ocular lenses.

Feeding the AGEs

Foods that are typically cooked at very high temperatures for longer than usual periods of time will induce high glycotoxins in the diet. One study showed that diabetics on a high glycotoxin diet showed a 50 to 100% increase in glycotoxins in their blood and urine compared to the group consuming a low glycotoxin diet. The group on the high glycotoxin diet also showed elevated levels of C-reactive protein, tumor necrosis factor (TNF) and other inflammatory markers. The group on the low glycotoxin diet showed reduced levels of harmful substances such as C-reactive protein and the bad cholesterol LDL.

So what can we do? Avoid foods that are deep-fried, seared, roasted and toasted. Likewise, limit baked goods with golden crusts and caramelization of sugars found in butterscotch and toffees. Instead, choose foods that are bathed in moisture, using cooking methods including stewing, steaming, and slow roasting in a low

Daily AGEs consumption in the standard Western diet is at least three times higher than the safety limit, which could partially explain the increase in chronic disease.[1]

temperature oven, dutch oven or crock pot. The important thing is to cook your food at temperatures well below the boiling point of water.

Free radical damage

In diabetics, oxidative stress and high levels of free radicals cause extensive damage to the arteries throughout the body. Oxidative stress occurs when there is an imbalance between the body's production of free radicals and the body's ability to detoxify them and repair the damage. Again, we see this damaging association between inflammation and disease. Oxidative stress and inflammation are 'joined at the hip', with each contributing to the other. Consequently, it is important that those with diabetes understand their need for antioxidant therapy to help reduce oxidative stress in order to lower the risk of diabetic complications.

The body's ability to produce antioxidants is somewhat dependent on your genetic makeup and your exposure to environmental factors such as diet and smoking. Lack of exercise only exposes us to more free radicals. Although the body can produce its own antioxidants, it is rarely enough to neutralize all the free radicals to which we are exposed. Examples of antioxidants include vitamins C, E, Coenzyme Q10 and beta-carotene, as well as trace elements selenium, copper and zinc.

Type 2 diabetes: an auto-immune disorder

Diabetes mellitus is now classified as an autoimmune disorder. An autoimmune disease refers to a group of chronic illnesses that involve almost every organ in the human body. In many of these diseases, including diabetes, the body's immune system can become misdirected, attacking the very organs it was designed to protect.

Diabetes care from the Mayo Clinic:

- Choose healthy foods and maintain a healthy weight. Losing just 5 to 10% if you are overweight can make a big difference to blood sugar control. Eat lots of vegetables, fruits, whole grains, legumes and limit saturated fats.
- Get active and make physical activity part of your daily routine. Regular exercise can help prevent prediabetes and Type 2 diabetes. Vary your routine: run, walk, lift light weights and enjoy yoga. You will actually control blood sugar better than with aerobic exercise alone.
- Pay attention to your feet. Consult your doctor about cuts, blisters, sores and redness that do not heal by themselves.
- Keep blood pressure and cholesterol under control.
- Take care of your teeth. Brush at least twice daily, as those with diabetes are prone to gum infections.
- If you smoke: QUIT!
- Take stress seriously: learn coping skills.

Beta-sitosterols in the lab

Research shows anti-hyperglycemic properties of plant sterols for diabetic conditions. Some studies show that beta-sitosterol may, in fact, help with the symptoms of diabetes. Inflammation is common in this condition as well as associated health concerns like weight management issues and heart disease. Diabetes is not a simple or easy condition to treat, but studies look promising that antioxidants and beta-sitosterol may be helpful in assisting those with this disease.[2]

A major study showed that rats given beta-sitosterol orally had increased fasting insulin levels, decreased fasting glycemia and improved glucose tolerance; meaning beta-sitosterol normalized blood sugar levels and functions.[3]

Other studies conclude:

- Oral beta-sitosterol in the seeds of *Parkia* species dramatically brought down high blood sugar levels in hyper-glycemic rats. This effect was not shown in healthy rats.[4]
- Oral beta-sitosterol given to diabetic rats improved their diamine oxidase (DAO) levels. DAO is an enzyme essential for the degradation of histamine, and it is mainly produced in the small intestine. Those with diabetes, who have little or no DAO, experience a build-up of histamine, which produces similar symptoms as those found in people with airborne allergies. Beta-sitosterol helps to increase the DAO levels and improve symptoms.[4]
- Oral beta-sitosterol given to diabetic rats improved blood sugar levels and inhibited glucose-6-phosphatase (G-6-P). G-6-P is an enzyme that plays a key role in the regulation of blood glucose levels. The body's ability to control this enzyme may become impaired, especially as we age. If this situation transpires, G-6-P increases the release of glucose from the liver and facilitates glucose production, which is detrimental to those with diabetic mellitus.[5]

Label explanation

The label on the Immuno-Care® bottle includes a caution that diabetics should consult their physician prior to using Immuno-Care®. This instruction is due to the fact that Immuno-Care® may in certain cases (but not necessarily in all) lower insulin require-ments.

Consequently, if you are diabetic and taking Immuno-Care®, you are advised to monitor your blood sugars on a regular basis, and if appropriate, consult with your physician about adjusting your insulin intake to ensure that you do not overdose on your own insulin.

Make a commitment to managing your diabetes: the more knowledge you have, the better equipped you will be to control it and get the most out of every day.

---

[1] Vlassara H et al. Protection against loss of innate defenses in adulthood by low advanced glycation end products (AGE) intake: role of the antiinflammatory AGE receptor-1. *J Clin Endocrinol Metab.* 2009 Nov;94(11):4483-91.

[2] Gylling H et al. Cholesterol metabolism in type 1 diabetics. *Diabetes.* 2004 Sep; 53 (9).

[3] Ivorra MD et al. Antihyperglycemic and insulin-releasing effects of beta-sitosterol, 3-beta-D-glycoside and its aglycone beta-sitosterol. *Archives Int. Pharmacodynamics & Therapeutics.* 1988;296:224-231.

[4] Jamaluddin F et al. Hypoglycemic effect of *Parkia speciosa* seeds due to the synergistic action of beta-sitosterol and stigmasterol. *Food Chem.* 1994;49:339-345.

[5] Atta-ur-Rahman, Chaudhary MI. Recent discoveries in the chemistry of natural products. *Pure Appl Chem.* 1994;66(10/11):1967-1974.

CHAPTER **NINE**

Fibromyalgia and Chronic Fatigue

Fibromyalgia and chronic fatigue syndrome share a number of symptoms, and their names are often used interchangeably in medical litreature. Fibromyalgia (FM) is an often misunderstood – even unrecognized – disorder that causes widespread muscle pain and tenderness, which tends to come and go and move about the body.

Chronic fatigue syndrome (CFS) is much more than just being tired a lot. People with fibromyalgia/CFS are so run down that it interferes with their lives and can make it hard to function at all. Some people with fibromyalgia/CFS say they have trouble staying on top of their responsibilities at home and on the job, while others are severely disabled and even bedridden. Furthermore, they're not just dealing with extreme fatigue, but also with a wide range of other symptoms, including flu-like symptoms and chronic pain.

If you are confused about the difference between the syndromes, you are not alone. Doctors are even confused. Many experts think that fibromyalgia and CFS may be variations of the same disease.

First surfacing in the 80s, the syndromes were portrayed as the 'yuppie flu', and were relatively rare conditions affecting mostly upper middle class, white professionals. Now researchers are shattering that image, as studies show that millions of North Americans may suffer from these syndromes. (And the majority of sufferers are not 'yuppies'.) It now spreads its ugly tentacles to all types of society, with no barriers to rich or poor. It has been marginalized and misunderstood for many years, and now medical science has defined it as a definite immune disorder of the modern era.

The American College of Rheumatology has developed a diagnosis and protocol that links many of the symptoms of FM to rheumatic-type conditions. Typical symptoms are pain in the muscles and joints. It is also associated with poor sleep and depression. Stress or lack of sleep tends to make the condition worse. More women suffer from this condition than men, and it is becoming all too common.

Fibromyalgia is thought to be traced to an injury, or a physical or emotional trauma, while CFS seems to be related to a flu-like onset.

> My husband's fibromyalgia has stopped him (and me) from sleeping for the past 6 years! Four days on Immuno-Care® and he was sleeping through the night. Now after almost 2 weeks, he is a changed person.
>
> A., Regina, SK

Central sensitization

After years of research, experts now suspect that something called 'central sensitization' is at least partially to blame for FM/CFS, and why they share many of the same features. Central sensitization relates to hypersensitivity of the central nervous system. People with fibromyalgia and CFS typically are more sensitive to bright light, chemicals, non-refreshing sleep, and difficulty concentrating. Various tissues also respond in a hypersensitive manner, including skin, muscle tissue and the lungs. This is why some doctors palpate or put pressure on certain parts of these patients to try to identify the sensitive areas of their bodies, and tests like the 18 point 'tender point' examination may help identify CFS and fibromyalgia.

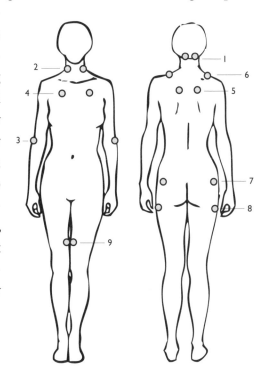

Tender points

Tender points are bilateral (both sides of body):

1. Occiput: back of neck where the base of the skull meets the neck

2. Low cervical region: front of the neck

3. Lateral epicondyle: near the crease of the elbow toward outer side of arm

4. Second rib: a few inches below the collarbone

5. Trapezius muscle: upper back; midway between the edge of the shoulder and the bottom of the neck

6. Supraspinatus muscle: shoulder

7. Gluteal: (rear end) at upper outer area of the buttocks

8. Greater trochanter: rear hip, at the bottom of the lower back

9. Knee: the inside of each knee pad

The first credible evidence of a biological basis for fibromyalgia/CFS came in 2006, when 20 researchers from different specialties each linked the illness with genes involved in the sympathetic nervous system and the HPA axis. These genes control how your body responds to things like injuries and stress.

Many researchers believe at least some cases of fibromyalgia/CFS are caused by an abnormal reaction to common infectious agents. The condition is tentatively linked to the Epstein-Barr virus, enteroviruses, human herpes virus 6 (HHV-6) and Lyme disease, although studies haven't proved a consistent causal link.

Multiple studies suggest, however, that the immune system may be chronically active in people with FM/CFS, which could at least partially explain the fatigue and lack of energy: in simple terms, your body *thinks* it's fighting an infection, whether it is or not, and that takes a lot of energy.

How plant sterols help

Plant sterols may indeed be very helpful in creating immune balance for those suffering with CFS and fibromyalgia. These rheumatic-type autoimmune diseases usually have inflammation in the form of Inter-

> I am writing to thank you with all my heart for giving my mother your wonderful product. She took 2 pills per day for the first week and then continued with one pill per day. In the short time span of 10 days, she has had a wonderful improvement and your supplement is the sole source of change that she made in her life. She is so excited that she wants to tell the world and distribute your product to everyone suffering from fibromyalgia.
>
> *R.M., California*

leukin-6 at their core, which can lead to pain. Phytosterols may inhibit the production of inflammatory IL-6. Research shows that Enzogenol™ also reduces the free radicals that can contribute to the development of muscle pain and fatigue disorders. Both are available in Immuno-Care®.

Antioxidants

Initial research has indicated a link between FM and oxidative stress. In a study involving 85 women suffering from primary fibromyalgia, researchers used malondialdehyde (the toxic metabolite of lipid peroxidation) to determine oxidative damage in the body. Tender points were stressed by palpation. Age, smoking, body mass index, and duration of disease were recorded.[1]

Malondialdehyde levels were significantly higher in the fibromyalgia patients than in the control group. It was shown that oxidant/antioxidant balances were changed in fibromyalgia patients. Age, smoking or duration of the disease did not appear to be significant factors. Researchers concluded that free radical levels may be responsible for the development of FM. Initial studies appear to support the hypothesis of FM as an oxidative disorder.

Likewise, in the case of CFS, a study by Italian researchers indicated oxidative damage to DNA and lipids in muscle specimens of CFS patients as compared to age-matched

> I would highly recommend Immuno-Care® for everyone who is struggling with fibromyalgia, depression, insomnia and other related illness. It has turned my life around and given me the opportunity to enjoy the life I had always enjoyed. If you are struggling with similar symptoms, I would highly recommend this product.
>
> T.Z., Saskatchewan, SK

controls.[2] Significantly, researchers at University of Canterbury showed DNA damage reduction as measured by the comet assay in general when diets were supplemented with Enzogenol™ and vitamin C.[3]

Immuno-Care® contains both a high concentration of sterols and also a broad spectrum antioxidant. It has been found to significantly alleviate the symptoms of fibromyalgia and CFS in a number of cases.

> I have been dealing with chronic fatigue and weakness for the past 6 months. My doctor recommended I take Immuno-Care®. While I am still working towards optimum health, I have noticed a marked increase in my energy level and well being while taking Immuno-Care®. I am grateful that there is a natural product to help me through this experience and have recommended Immuno-Care® to family and friends. I am happily off the couch and doing more to take care of my family and lead a more normal life. Thank you!
>
> *L.D., Ontario*

---

[1] Bagis S, Tamer L et al. Free radicals and antioxidants in primary fibromyalgia: an oxidative stress disorder? *Rheumatol Int.* 2005 Apr;25(3):188-90.

[2] Fulle S, Mecocci P et al. Specific oxidative alterations in vastus lateralis muscle of patients with the diagnosis of chronic fatigue syndrome. *Free Radic Biol Med.* 2000 Dec 15;29(12):1252-9.

[3] Senthilmohan ST, Zhang J, Stanley RA. Effects of flavonoid extract Enzogenol® with vitamin C on protein oxidation and DNA damage in older human subjects. *Nutr Res.* 2003;(23):1199-1210.

CHAPTER **TEN**

Heart Disease

Thank goodness we are finally becoming aware that heart disease is the number one killer of both men and women. While the statistic is frightening on the surface, there is much we can do to protect our heart health, and we can address many of the factors contributing to heart disease – including high cholesterol, and elevated homocysteine and C-reactive protein – through lifestyle changes, including diet, exercise and nutritional supplements. Let's look at each of them in turn.

High cholesterol: a snapshot

High cholesterol doesn't discriminate: people of all ages and backgrounds can and do get high cholesterol and, throughout the world, blood cholesterol levels vary widely. Generally, people who live in countries where blood cholesterol levels are lower, such as Japan, have lower rates of heart disease. Countries with very high cholesterol levels, such as Finland and Ireland, have very high rates of coronary heart disease. However, some populations with similar total cholesterol levels have very different heart disease rates, suggesting that other factors also influence risk for coronary heart disease.

High cholesterol is more common in men younger than 55 years and in women older than 55 years. The risk for high cholesterol increases with age.

North America's cholesterol burden:

- Approximately one in every six adults in the United States (16.3% of the U.S. adult population) has high total cholesterol. High total cholesterol is defined as 240 mg/dL (milligrams per decilitre) and above.
- People with high total cholesterol have approximately twice the risk of heart disease as people with optimal levels. A desirable level is lower than 200 mg/dL.
- For adult Americans, the average level is about 200 mg/dL, which is borderline high risk.
- Now, more women than men have high cholesterol in the United States.

According to Statistics Canada, over 40% of Canadians aged 20 to 79 have an unhealthy level of total cholesterol and about 25% have an unhealthy level of triglycerides. As you can see, high blood cholesterol leading to heart disease is a major concern, and should be taken seriously.

The skinny on cholesterol
Despite its bad press, we actually need cholesterol, a wax-like steroid molecule that plays a critical role in metabolism. It is a major component of cellular membranes, where its concentration varies depending on the function of the particular cell. For example, the membrane of liver cells contains fairly large fractions of cholesterol (approximately 30%).

The cholesterol in cell membranes serves two primary functions. First, it modulates the fluidity of membranes, allowing them to maintain their function over a wide range of temperatures. Second, it prevents leakage of ions (molecules used by the cell to interact with its environment) by acting as a cellular insulator.[1] This effect is critical for the proper function of neuronal cells. The cholesterol-rich myelin sheath insulates neurons and allows them to transmit electrical impulses rapidly over distances.

Cholesterol has other important roles in human metabolism: it serves as a precursor to the steroid hormones, which include the sex hormones (androgens and estrogens); mineral-corticoids, which control the balance of water and minerals in the kidney, and glucocorticoids, which control protein and carbohydrate metabolism, immune suppression, and inflammation. Cholesterol is also the precursor to vitamin D. Likewise, cholesterol provides the framework for the synthesis of bile acids, which emulsify dietary fats for absorption. In fact, cholesterol is naturally present in cell walls or membranes everywhere in the body, including the brain, nerves, muscles, skin, liver, intestines, and heart. It takes only a small amount of cholesterol in the blood, however, to meet these needs.

LDL and HDL

LDL (low density lipoprotein) cholesterol can build up on the walls of your arteries and increase your chances of getting heart disease. That is why LDL cholesterol is referred to as 'bad' cholesterol. The lower your LDL cholesterol number, the lower your risk.

When it comes to high-density lipoprotein (HDL) cholesterol – otherwise known as 'good' cholesterol – the higher the number, the lower your risk. Some people refer to HDL as your insurance factor against heart disease. This is because HDL cholesterol protects against heart disease by taking the 'bad' cholesterol out of your blood and keeping it from building up in your arteries.

Healthy levels of lipids in blood

Total cholesterol	< 4.5 mmol/L (6 to 19 years)[1] < 5.2 mmol/L (20 to 79 years)[1]
Triglycerides	< 1.7 mmol/L[1]
Low density lipoprotein-cholesterol LDL, 'bad' cholesterol	< 3.4 mmol/L[2]
High density lipoprotein-cholesterol HDL, 'good' cholesterol	> 1.0 mmol/L men[1] > 1.3 mmol/L women[1]
Ratio of total cholesterol to HDL cholesterol (TC/HDL-C)	< 4.11[2]

Based on recommendations from the CHMS Physician Advisory Committee, and updated 2010 StatsCan.ca

More about lipoproteins

Emerging research into underappreciated aspects of cholesterol biochemistry has revealed that levels of cholesterol account for only a portion of the cardiovascular risk profile. Particles responsible for transporting cholesterol through the blood, known as lipoproteins, offer important insights into the development of atherosclerosis.

In fact, the size and density of lipoproteins are important factors for cardiovascular risk: for example, large, buoyant LDL particles are much less dangerous than small, dense LDL particles; likewise large, buoyant HDL particles offer greater vascular protection than smaller, more dense HDL.

The development of advanced lipid testing strategies that take the importance of lipoprotein particle size into consideration, such as the Vertical Auto Profile (VAP) or Nuclear Magnetic Resonance (NMR), allow a far deeper assessment of cardiovascular risk than a conventional lipid profile utilized by most mainstream medical practitioners.

Furthermore, metabolic processes, such as oxidation and glycation, modify the functionality of lipoproteins, transforming them from cholesterol transport vehicles into highly reactive molecules capable of damaging the delicate endothelial cells that line our arterial walls.

To get a sense of what oxidation refers to, imagine an iron pipe lying on the ground. As it weathers from years of rain, environmental exposure, sun, and other factors, it begins to rust. The rust is caused by oxidation. Likewise, in your body, free oxygen radicals are created during normal metabolism. These free radicals are missing a simple electron and are in search of another molecule that they can combine with to become whole.

In effect, your body is 'rusting' as it goes through its lifetime, with free oxygen radicals wildly running through your system, searching for a mate. The more free radicals your body contains, the more damage that's likely to be done. The best way to see this damage is through our normal aging process. Ingesting antioxidants is a means of reducing this process, as they donate an electron and stop the progress of the free radical.

Glycation, on the other hand, is a process in which sugar and protein molecules combine to form a tangled mass of tissue. Glycated tissue is tough and inflexible, leading to wrinkling not only of the skin, but also of important internal organs.

This endothelial damage both initiates and promotes the beginning of plaque formation in the arteries, or atherogenesis. Scientifically supported, natural interventions can target the formation of these modified lipoproteins and help avert deadly cardiovascular diseases such as heart attack and stroke.

Triglycerides

Triglycerides are storage lipids that have a critical role in metabolism and energy production; they provide your body with denser sources of energy than carbohydrates, which make them superior for long-term energy storage. (While glucose is the preferred energy source for most cells, it is a bulky molecule that contains little energy for the amount of space it occupies. Glucose is primarily stored in the liver and muscles as glycogen. The average human can only store enough glucose in the liver for about 12 hours worth of energy without food, but can store enough fat to power the body for significantly longer.)

Cholesterol, on the other hand, is used to build cells and certain hormones. Because triglycerides and cholesterol can't dissolve in blood, they circulate throughout your body with the help of proteins that transport the lipids (lipoproteins). High levels of triglycerides have been associated with a higher risk of heart disease. Triglycerides provide unique information as markers associated with the risk for heart disease and stroke, especially when an individual also has low HDL cholesterol and elevated levels of LDL.

> 90% of Canadians have at least one risk factor for heart disease or stroke, including smoking, alcohol, physical inactivity, obesity, high blood pressure, high blood cholesterol, diabetes.
> *Heartandstroke.ca*

When cholesterol goes bad

If a person has too much cholesterol in the bloodstream, the excess may be deposited in arteries, including the coronary arteries of the heart, the carotid arteries to the brain, and the arteries that supply blood to the legs. Cholesterol deposits are a component of the plaques that cause narrowing and blockage of the arteries, producing signs and symptoms originating from the particular part of the body that has decreased blood supply.

Coronary heart disease (CHD) is caused by cholesterol and fat being deposited in the walls of the arteries that supply nutrients and oxygen to the heart. Like any muscle, the heart needs a constant supply of oxygen and nutrients, which are carried to it by the blood in the coronary arteries. Narrowing of the arteries decreases that supply and can cause angina (chest pain) when the heart muscle does not receive enough oxygen. Cholesterol plaques can rupture, resulting in a blood clot formation that completely blocks the artery, stopping all blood flow and causing a heart attack, in which heart muscle cells die from lack of oxygen and nutrients.

Factors in high cholesterol

High cholesterol levels are due to a variety of factors including heredity and lifestyle. Less commonly, underlying conditions of the liver, thyroid, or kidney may affect blood cholesterol levels.

Heredity: Genes may influence how the body metabolizes LDL (bad) cholesterol. Familial hypercholesterolemia is an inherited form of high cholesterol that may lead to early heart disease.

Weight: Excess weight may modestly increase your LDL (bad) cholesterol level. Losing weight may lower LDL and raise HDL (good) cholesterol levels.

Physical activity/exercise: Regular physical activity may lower triglycerides and raise HDL cholesterol levels.

Age and sex: Before menopause, women usually have lower total cholesterol levels than men of the same age. As women and men age, their blood cholesterol levels rise until approximately 60 to 65 years of age. After about age 50, women often have higher total cholesterol levels than men of the same age. This may be a result of increased insulin resistance (a condition that contributes to the development of diabetes), which typically occurs after menopause and is associated with a higher level of triglycerides. In older women, then, levels of triglycerides provide an excellent indicator of coronary heart disease.

Mental stress: Several studies have shown that stress raises blood cholesterol levels over the long term. One way that stress may do this is by affecting your habits. For example, when some people are under stress, they console themselves by eating fatty foods – a factor in higher levels of blood cholesterol.

Fat facts

Despite what those diet fads of days gone by might have led you to believe, dietary fats are necessary to promote optimal health. The trick is to eat the right fats, particularly when it comes to cholesterol.

Unsaturated fats are called good fats, for example, because they can improve blood cholesterol levels, ease inflammation, stabilize heart rhythms, and play a number of other beneficial roles. Unsaturated fats are predominantly found in foods from plants, such as vegetable oils, nuts, and seeds, as well as marine sources like fish. They are liquids at room temperature.

Saturated fatty acids, on the other hand, have all the hydrogen that the carbon atoms can hold. Saturated fats are usually solid at room temperature and they are more stable; that is, they do not combine readily with oxygen. Saturated fatty acids are the main dietary culprit in raising blood cholesterol. The main sources of saturated fatty acids in the typical American diet are foods such as beef, beef fat, veal, lamb, pork, lard, poultry fat, butter, cream, milk, cheeses and other dairy products made from whole milk. (These foods also contain dietary cholesterol, the impact of which is explained below.) Foods from plants that contain high amounts of saturated fatty acids include coconut oil, palm oil and palm kernel oil (often called tropical oils) and cocoa butter.

Trans-fats occur naturally in some animal-based foods, but most of our dietary exposure to them occurs in products made with artificially created semi-solid fats like shortening and hard margarine. Also known as hydrogenated fats, these fats are made by adding hydrogen to a liquid fat and adding pressure. Trans-fats provide a double-whammy when it comes to cholesterol: not only do trans-fats increase plasma levels of LDL cholesterol, but they also reduce plasma levels of HDL cholesterol and increase the blood level of atherogenic lipoprotein. This suggests that trans-fatty acids may be a greater risk factor for CHD than dietary saturated fatty acids. Eliminate these fats from your diet!

Cholesterol is another lipid found in animal sources of food. Despite common per-

Nutritious, delicious coconut oil

While a source of saturated fat, coconut oil contains medium-chain triglycerides (MCT). MCT are easily digested and absorbed sources of fuel, associated with suppressed body fat accumulation.

ception, however, evidence indicates that dietary cholesterol is not a major factor influencing plasma cholesterol and lipoprotein levels in the general population. It appears that the earlier predictions of the effect of each 100 mg of dietary cholesterol on plasma total cholesterol were too high (namely, 1.75 mmol/L for each 100 mg/day dietary cholesterol).

All the meta-analyses and carefully controlled studies reported since 1993 estimate that a decrease of 100 mg dietary cholesterol results in a decrease of plasma cholesterol of 0.05 mmol/L. On a population basis, this change is relatively insignificant considering that it represents approximately 1% of the average population plasma cholesterol concentration. In other words, dietary cholesterol doesn't create a huge increase in blood cholesterol levels for most people. Of course, there is evidence that some individuals may be high responders to dietary cholesterol, but the effect appears to be primarily on plasma total cholesterol; the effect of dietary cholesterol on plasma LDL varies.

Alternatively, there is appreciable scientific support for the benefits of reducing the intakes of dietary saturated and trans-fats in lowering the risk of CHD. Guidelines for the prevention of CHD should therefore, focus primarily on reducing the dietary intakes of saturated and trans-fats. Health Canada proposes a health claim stating that diets low in saturated and trans-fats may reduce the risk of heart disease.

Focus your dietary fat intake on polyunsaturated fatty acids from fish and plant sources, like olive oil, walnut oil and other plant-based oils, as well as nuts and seeds, to support healthy cholesterol levels.

C-reactive protein

Along with cholesterol, C-reactive protein (CRP) is a factor in heart disease risk. CRP is a marker of inflammation, and is elevated in the blood when there is widespread inflammation in the body. The evidence now available indicates that inflammation and molecules such as CRP associated with inflammation may be as important as cholesterol in determining the development of atherosclerosis (hardening of the arteries) and heart disease.

C-reactive protein is produced by the liver in response to the pro-inflammatory cytokine Interleukin-6.[2] However, CRP is not merely a nonspecific marker of inflammation and atherosclerosis. It actively participates in lesion formation through induction of endothelial dysfunction and leukocyte activation.[3,4] Some researchers have suggested that a chronic infection with certain bacteria or viruses may also play a part in raising the CRP.

Elevated levels of C-reactive protein are now associated with increased risk of heart attack and death from heart disease. People whose CRP levels are in the upper third of the population have double the risk of a heart attack of people with lower CRP levels. Women are now as susceptible as men for CVD, in fact maybe even more so. CRP and other inflammatory markers should be considered in the prediction of cardiovascular disease in women.[5]

Inflammation likely contributes to heart disease by teaming up with the LDL cholesterol, which is deposited in the plaques that adhere to blood vessel walls and impede blood flow. The inflammatory process may damage these plaques, allowing tiny portions of plaque to break off into the bloodstream. These small fragments of plaque can then be swept away to lodge in small blood vessels in the heart or brain, causing a heart attack or stroke.

Since C-reactive protein is a gauge of inflammation, a test that measures CRP is valuable. One such test is known as the high-sensitivity CRP assay (hs-CRP). Many doctors now believe that it is important to measure hs-CRP levels along with cholesterol to determine the risk of heart disease and to evaluate disease progression and prognosis in those who already have cardiovascular disease.[5]

To be precise, hs-CRP levels under 1.0 milligram per litre, or mg/L, carry a low risk of developing heart disease. Levels between 1.0 mg/L and 3.0 mg/L are associated with an average risk. And hs-CRP levels over 3.0 mg/L carry a high risk for cardiovascular disease.

People with inflammatory diseases such as rheumatoid arthritis or lupus can also have markedly elevated C-reactive protein levels.[6] Other causes of high CRP include cancer, trauma, burns, and recent major surgery. CRP can raise a thousandfold higher than normal from severe inflammation. In cases of extremely high C-reactive protein levels due to inflammatory diseases, the prognostic value of CRP as a cardiac risk factor cannot be accurately determined.

Gender matters: heart disease risk in women

Heart disease is the leading cause of death among women – and one of the most preventable. Research is giving us insights into how we can control the risk.

We've come a long way since the days when a woman's worry over heart disease centered exclusively on its threat to the men in her life. We now know it's not just a man's problem. Every year, the leading cause of death in North America is coronary heart disease, claiming women and men in nearly equal numbers, and totalling about 500,000 lives. More than 6.5 million women have some form of CHD. Of those who survive a heart attack, 46% will be disabled by heart failure within six years. The statistics below are quoted from the *Women's Heart Foundation*:

- 42% of women who have heart attacks die within one year, compared to 24% of men.
- Under age 50, women's heart attacks are twice as likely as men's to be fatal.
- Heart attacks kill six times as many women as breast cancer.

At-risk:
- 71% of women experience early warning signs of heart attack with sudden onset of extreme weakness that feels like the flu and often with no chest pain at all.
- Nearly two-thirds of the deaths from heart attacks in women occur among those who have no history of chest pain.
- Smoking, diabetes and abnormal blood lipids erase a woman's estrogen protection.
- Women who smoke risk having a heart attack 19 years earlier than non-smoking women.
- Women with diabetes have more than double the risk of heart attack than non-diabetic women. Diabetes doubles the risk of a second heart attack in women but not in men. Diabetes affects many more women than men after the age of 45.
- Marital stress worsens the prognosis in women with heart disease.

Compared to men:
- Men's plaque distributes in clumps whereas women's plaque distributes more evenly throughout artery walls. This results

in women's angiographic studies being misinterpreted as 'normal.'

- Women wait longer than men to go to an emergency room when having a heart attack and physicians are slower to recognize the presence of heart attacks in women because characteristic patterns of chest pain and EKG changes are less frequently present.

- Women are twice as likely as men to die within the first few weeks after suffering a heart attack.

- 46% of women and 22% of men who have survived a heart attack will be disabled with heart failure within six years.

- Women between the ages of 40-59 are up to four times more likely to die from heart bypass surgery than men the same age.

- Studies show women who are eligible candidates to receive life-saving, clot-buster drugs are far less likely than men to receive them.

- Women's hearts respond better than men's to healthy lifestyle changes.

The *New England Journal of Medicine* reports that it is very important for women to get all associated markers tested for cardiovascular disease risk. In one study, prediction models that incorporated markers of inflammation in addition to lipids were significantly better at predicting risk than models based on lipid levels alone (P<0.001).

The levels of hs-CRP and serum amyloid A were significant predictors of risk even in the subgroup of women with LDL cholesterol levels below 130 mg per decilitre (3.4 mmol per litre), the target for primary prevention established by the *National Cholesterol Education Program*.

Vitamin C reduces C-reactive protein

A *University of California at Berkeley* study showed participants who started out with C-reactive protein levels greater than 2.00 mg/L and received 1000 mg per day vitamin C, had 34% lower levels of CRP compared with the placebo group after only two months.[7,8] This study was done based on previous findings that vitamin C supplements reduce elevated CRP.

A healthy diet significantly reduces C-reactive protein

Eating too much saturated fat or high-glycemic carbohydrates increases C-reactive protein.[9,10] One study showed a 39% decrease in CRP levels after only eight weeks of consuming a diet low in saturated fat and cholesterol.[11] The study participants also saw reductions in their LDL, total cholesterol, body weight, and arterial stiffness.

Another study showed that eating cholesterol-lowering food works about as well as consuming a very low-fat diet plus statin drug therapy. This study showed a 33.3% reduction in C-reactive protein and 30.9% reduction in LDL in subjects eating a very low-fat diet and taking a statin drug. Those who ate the cholesterol-lowering foods showed a 28.2% reduction in CRP and a 28.6% reduction in LDL. This study showed that participants eating cholesterol-lowering foods achieved almost the same benefit as those who followed a very low-fat diet and took a statin drug.

The cholesterol-lowering foods used in this study included almonds, soy protein, fibre, and plant sterols. Few people can follow a rigorous low-fat diet and some people want to avoid statin drugs. Based on the results of this study, those who need to reduce LDL and/or CRP blood levels will benefit from eating cholesterol-lowering foods or taking supplements such as soluble fibre powder before heavy meals.[12]

Another study of 3,920 people found that subjects who ingested the most dietary fibre had a 41% lower risk of elevated CRP levels, compared with those who ate the least fibre. The doctors who conducted this study concluded that fibre intake is independently associated with serum CRP concentration and support the recommendation of a diet with a high fibre content."[13]

The important take-home lesson for those with high C-reactive protein levels that persist even after initiating statin drug therapy is that, you may be able to achieve significant added benefits by making dietary modifications, taking at least 1,000 mg of vitamin C each day, and following other proven ways to quell chronic inflammatory reactions.

> Seven out of 10 children (ages four to eight) and half of adults do not eat the recommended daily minimum of five servings of vegetables and fruit.
> *Heartandstroke.ca*

Although C-reactive protein is a general, nonspecific marker of inflammation, the bottom line is that it is useful in helping predict the risk of heart disease and stroke. All women face the threat of heart disease. But becoming aware of symptoms and risks unique to women, as well as eating a heart-healthy diet and exercising, can help protect you. (Men too!)

Homocysteine and your heart

Homocysteine is an abnormal protein created when a specific amino acid called methionine is metabolized, usually as a by-product of consuming meat. In most people, homocysteine is quickly cleared out of the arteries and therefore, does not create a problem. However, for some people, homocysteine is not efficiently cleared out and can pose significant health risks.

If unhealthy levels of homocysteine accumulate in the blood, the delicate lining of an artery (endothelium) can be damaged. Homocysteine can both initiate and potentiate atherosclerosis. For example, homocysteine-induced injury to the arterial wall is one of the factors that can initiate the process of atherosclerosis, leading to endothelial dysfunction and eventually to heart attacks and strokes.

Homocysteine and congestive heart failure

Small clinical studies have shown that patients with congestive heart failure (CHF) suffer from elevated plasma homocysteine levels. [14] Based on preclinical evidence that the myocardium may be especially susceptible to homocysteine-induced injury and on observations linking homocysteine to oxidative stress and ventricular remodelling, it has been hypothesized that elevated plasma homocysteine levels would increase the risk of CHF. [15,16,17]

Accordingly, researchers investigated the relationship of plasma homocysteine concentration to the risk of CHF in a community-based sample of adults (2491 adults, mean age 72 years including 1547 women who were free of CHF or prior myocardial infarction at baseline). This was the well-known *Framingham Heart Study* during the 1979-1982 and 1986-1990 examination periods. In one study that examined patients without any manifestation of coronary heart disease at baseline, investigators found that the association of plasma homocysteine levels with risk of CHF was maintained in men and women, and concluded "an increased plasma homocysteine level independently predicts risk of the development of CHF in adults without prior myocardial infarction."

Causes of elevated homocysteine

Studies have shown that high levels of homocysteine are caused by a lack of nutrients in the diet, particularly the B group of vitamins. Without these essential vitamins, your body is unable to produce the enzymes necessary to remove homocysteine efficiently from your blood. Homocysteine will cause damage to your arteries when present in high concentrations, hence the link between homocysteine and heart disease.

Fortunately, in the late 60's, Dr. Kilmer McCully determined through extensive research that taking adequate amounts of folic acid (vitamin B9), along with vitamins B6 and B12, will normalize levels of homocysteine.

Make sure you get a homocysteine test as part of your next visit to the doctor, or on your own at a licensed medical facility. A homocysteine test, along with the other blood tests, may help establish your risk of developing heart disease.

Healthy homocysteine levels

The normal level of homocysteine in the average healthy person should be 5 to 15 micro mol/L. The optimal level of homocysteine in your blood would be under 7 micro mol/L.

Plant sterols and your heart

Dietary plant sterols are known to reduce plasma cholesterol levels and thereby reduce cardiovascular risk. Recent observations from animal and human studies have demonstrated anti-inflammatory effects of phytosterols. For example, several animal and human studies report reductions in the levels of proinflammatory cytokines, including C-reactive protein, after consumption of dietary plant sterols.[18]

A randomised, double-blind study of Immuno-Care® on humans conducted at the *Human Nutraceutical Research Unit* at the University of Guelph, Ontario showed:

"Immuno-Care® supplement is effective in reducing circulating levels of LDL cholesterol and increasing circulating levels of HDL cholesterol. It is of interest to note that there was a significant decrease in the ratio of TC/HDL, and in the ratio of LDL/HDL cholesterol in the Immuno-Care® group. A decrease in these ratios corresponds to an associated decrease in cardiovascular disease (CVD) risk, because these ratios are markers for a reduction in the risk of developing atherosclerosis. Consequently these results would be of considerable benefit to the health of hypercolesterolemic individuals at risk of developing CVD."

Immuno-Care® showed promise at lower levels of plant sterols per day than what was typically used in other studies. The dosage used was a loading dose of two capsules per day for seven days, then the control group was reduced to one capsule in the morning for the remainder of the study. Enteric coating plays an important part in protecting these nutrients from stomach acids, which tend to reduce the amount of beta-sitosterol entering the small intestine. Antioxidants in Immuno-Care® also play a role in reducing inflammation and oxidative damage.

---

[1] Sterols Reduce Proton and Sodium leaks through Lipid Bilayers. Haines T.H. Prog. Lipid Res. 40(4) Jul 2001

[2] C-Reactive Protein, Interleukin-6 and Fibrogen as Predictors of Coronary Heart Disease. The Prime Study. Luc, Bard etal. *Art Throm Vasc Biol* 2003;23:1255.

[3] Hotline editorial. *European Heart Journal*, 2001,22 349-35

[4] Direct Pro-inflammatory Effect of C-reactive Protein on Human Endothelial Cells. Pasceri, James et al. *Circulation* 2000:102:2165.

[5] C-reactive Protein and other markers of inflammation in the Prediction of Cardiovacular Disease in Women. Ridker P, Hennekens C. et al, *N Engl J Med*, March 23, 2000, Volume 342 No. 1.

[6] Serum C-reactive protein levels in disease such as rheumatoid arthritis. Morley JJ, Kushner I. et al. *Ann N Y, Acad Sci*. 1982, 389: 406-418.

[7] Vitamin C treatment reduces elevated C-reactive protein. Block G, Jensen CD, Dalvi TB, et al. *Free Radic Biol Med*. 2009 Jan 1;46(1):70-7.

[8] Available at: http://berkeley.edu/news/media/releases/2008/11/12 vitaminc.shtml

[9] Relationships between serum fatty acid composition and multiple markers of inflammation and endothelial function in an elderly population. Petersson H et al *Atherosclerosis*. 2008 Jul 1.

[10] Dietary glycemic index, dietary glycemic load, blood lipids, and C-reactive protein. Levitan EB et al. *Metabolism*. 2008 Mar;57(3):437.

[11] Effects of a dietary portfolio of cholesterol-lowering foods vs lovastatin on serum lipids and C-reactive protein. Jenkins DJ et al. *JAMA*. 2003 Jul 23;290(4):502-10.

[12] Attenuation of inflammation with short-term dietary intervention is associated with a reduction of arterial stiffness in subjects with hypercholesterolaemia. Pirro M et al. *Eur J Cardiovasc Prev Rehabil*. 2004 Dec;11(6):497-502.

[13] Dietary fiber and C-reactive protein: findings from national health and nutrition examination survey data. Ajani UA et al. *J Nutr*. 2004 May;134(5):1181-5.

[14] Plasma atherogenic markers in congestive heart failure and post transplant (heart)patients, Cooke G, J. Am. Coll Cardiol. 2000;36:509-516.

[15] Plasma Homocysteine and Risk for Congestive Heart Failure in Adults Without Prior Myocardial Infarction. Vasan, Beiser et al. *JAMA*. 2003;289:1251-1257.

[16] The oxidant stress of hyperhomocyst(e)inemia. (editorial). Loscalzo J et al, *J. Clin. Invest.* 1996;98:5-7

[17] Homocyteine linked to left cardiac ventricle remodeling, Blacher et al. *Am J Physiol Heart Circ. Physiol* 2003; 285: H679-H686.

[18] Beyond cholesterol-lowering effects of plant sterols: clinical and experimental evidence of anti-inflammatory properties, Othman RA, Moghadasian MH, *Nutr Rev*. 2011, Jul;69(7):371-82.

CHAPTER **ELEVEN**

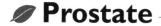 # Prostate

The majority of men older than 50 years will be affected by benign (non-cancerous) prostatic hyperplasia (BPH), better known as enlargement of the prostate gland. When the prostate gland enlarges, it presses on the urethra (the tube that transports urine and semen to the outside of the body). Even the smallest increase in the size of the prostate gland can compress the urethra.

Symptoms of BPH differ among patients, but certain symptoms occur in the majority of cases. The number and intensity of symptoms also vary with age. The most commonly reported symptoms of BPH include:

- Increased frequency in urinating during the day
- Need to urinate several times during the night
- Sensation of needing to urinate immediately
- Dribbling urine or having difficulty stopping urination
- Having the feeling of still needing to urinate even after the stream has stopped
- Pain or a burning sensation during urination
- Complete retention of urine: in advanced BPH, the enlarged prostate can completely obstruct the passage of urine.

BPH occurs because testosterone combines with an enzyme called 5-alpha-reductase to produce another hormone called dihydrotestosterone (DHT). DHT triggers prostate enlargement. To treat BPH, conventional medicine usually focuses on drugs that inhibit the hormones that control prostate growth or that relax the smooth muscles inside the prostate gland, including alpha-receptor blocking agents and 5-alpha-reductase inhibitors. Surgery is also a treatment option. However, most men can benefit from a variety of complementary nutritional strategies that offer proven relief for BPH.

Likewise, remedies derived from plants are widely used for this purpose in Europe.

Clinical studies show that beta-sitosterol, a major component of Immuno-Care®, is one of the most effective plant-derived options available for BPH. A multi-centric, placebo-controlled, double-blind clinical trial of beta-sitosterol for the treatment of BPH proved what a powerful supplement beta-sitosterol is for BPH.[1] This randomized study involved 177 patients with benign prostatic hyperplasia and was designed to assess the safety and efficacy of using beta-sitosterol in treating this condition.

> I can attest from personal experience that Immuno-Care® is far and away the most effective product on the market for increasing urine flow and reducing nighttime visits to the bathroom: in my case, generally reduced from four visits a night to two. This has made a great difference in the quality of my sleep, and also my alertness the following day. As a side benefit, I have had a considerable reduction in the frequency of flu and colds, and also a thickening of my hair.
>
> *A.F., Calgary, Alberta*

Over the six month duration of the study, individuals in the treatment group received 130 mg of beta-sitosterol daily. Parameters used to monitor the effectiveness of this treatment approach included peak urinary flow rate (Qmax), post-void residual volume (PVR) and qualitative determinators provided by the International Prostate Symptom Scores (IPSS); and changes in the quality of life index value.

Researchers found statistically significant results over the placebo group: Qmax values increased by 44%, while PVR values improved by 53%, after adjustment for placebo effects. Quality of life scores and IPSS values also showed a statistically significant improvement. These results indicate that beta-sitosterol is, in fact, an effective treatment option for individuals with BPH.

The dose of 130 mg beta-sitosterol per day has been confirmed in practice by almost 15 years of empirical experience, and is fully within the registered dose range of the BPH indication in Germany.

Similar results occurred in a trial organized by the *Prostate Help Association* in the UK, which included 100 participants. The trial showed:[2]

- After 3 weeks, 75% of the participants had an average 23% improvement in IPSS scores
- After 8 weeks, 83% of the participants showed an average 33% improvement of IPSS scores
- After 12 weeks, 90% of the participants recorded an average 44% improvement in IPSS scores.

Other studies:

- BPH symptoms improved significantly in only 45 days with beta-sitosterol content extract of saw palmetto. Of the 505 patients studied, 90% had improvement in 90 days. The study shows that plant sterols inhibit 5-alpha-reductase, which prevents testosterone from being converted to DHT. This multicentre, open study was carefully and precisely carried out and proves beyond doubt the safety and effectiveness of beta-sitosterol in the treatment of BPH.[3]

- A double-blind, randomized study compared finasteride (Proscar), a drug frequently prescribed to increase urinary flow, with a plant extract containing saw palmetto whose active ingredient is beta-sitosterol. This study showed that both had a similar, positive effect on increasing urinary flow. The plant extract gave rise to fewer complaints of decreased libido and impotence, a common side effect of finasteride.[4, 5]

- Another study by *Habib et al* showed that the phytosterols in powerful saw palmetto extracts were very effective in treating BPH due to the anti-estrogenic activity of beta-sitosterol in prostatic tissue of BPH patients. The phytosterols also effectively inhibited the conversion of testosterone into dihydro testosterone by 5-alpha-reductase. Beta-sitosterol was believed to be responsible for blocking the activity of testosterone that was causing the swelling.[5]

A hair-raising fear
All men fear losing their hair. I used to hear people say that if your mother's father was bald, then there were good chances you also would be bald. Other old wives' tales suggest a link to

the hormone testosterone: whether too much or too little. Closer to the truth, studies show that some hair loss in men does seem to be tied to the hormone testosterone. When does having hair change to losing hair? And the answer is: when testosterone is converted to dihydrotestosterone (DHT).

Elevated DHT is associated with a low free testosterone

Going bald?
The same DHT process that leads to BPH also triggers hair loss in men. If you are losing your hair, be sure to schedule a prostate exam on your next doctor's visit. (In some cases a side effect of Immuno-Care® can be the growth/regrowth of hair. We have seen this in several alopecia patients.

---

level due to the fact that it has been converted to DHT. DHT was responsible for the growth of your prostate gland during puberty. Unfortunately, DHT can subsequently cause BPH and contribute to loss of hair.

Studies have shown that beta-sitosterol can inhibit the conversion of testosterone to DHT by inhibiting the production of the enzyme 5-alpha-reductase.[6] It is this enzyme that actually converts testosterone to DHT. Further, it is this enzyme, 5-alpha-reductase and its actions, which have been linked to male pattern hair loss.[6]

Immuno-Care® and prostate health
Phytosterols have been used extensively in Europe to alleviate symptoms of BPH. With Immuno-Care®, you can enjoy the same benefits.

[1] Klippel KF, Hiltl DM, Schipp B. A multicentric, placebo-controlled, double-blind clinical trial of beta-sitosterol (phytosterol) for the treatment of benign prostatic hyperplasia. *Br J Urol.* 1997 Sep;80(3):427-32.

[2] *Ibid.*

[3] Braeckman J. The extract of *Sereona repens* in the treatment of benign prostatic hyperplasia: a multicenter open study. *Current Therapeutic Research.* 1994 July;55(7):776-785.

[4] Carraro J et al. Comparison of phytotherapy (Permixon) with finasteride in the treatment of benign prostate hyperplasia: a randomized international study of 1,098 patients. *Prostate.* 1996 Oct;29(4):231-240.

[5] Habib FK et al. *Seronoa repens* (Permixon) inhibits the 5 alpha-reductase activity of human prostate cancer cell lines without interfering with PSA expression. *Int J Cancer.* 2005 Mar 20;114(2):190-4.

[6] Prager N et al. A randomized, double-blind, placebo-controlled trial to determine the effectiveness of botanically derived inhibitors of 5-alpha-reductase in the treatment of androgenetic alopecia. *J Altern Complement Med.* 2002 Apr; 8(2):143-52.

CHAPTER TWELVE
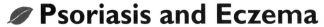 Psoriasis and Eczema

The Center for Disease Control (CDC) estimates that 150,000 people a year are diagnosed with psoriasis and the incidence of eczema is also increasing dramatically. These two conditions are very similar and it can be hard to tell them apart. In England alone, data suggests there was a 42% rise in diagnosis of eczema between 2001 and 2005, by which time it was estimated to affect 5.7 million adults and children. General practitioners' records of over 9 million patients were used by researchers to assess how many people had an inflammatory skin disorder. It showed that by 2005, one in nine of the population had, at some point, been affected by eczema. The highest rate was in boys aged between five and nine.

What's the difference?

Psoriasis and eczema are very similar in appearance and most people find it difficult to tell the difference. Both are characterized by red, scaly skin eruptions. In the case of eczema, the patient has dry red skin in the form of blisters that itch tremendously. In the case of psoriasis, the patient has raised red skin which is very rough and itches too.

Both the terms eczema and psoriasis are derived from Greek language. Psoriasis originates from the word *psoera*, which means 'to itch' while eczema means 'boil out.' Eczema and psoriasis generally attack people of different age groups. Eczema is known to be more prevalent in children than in adults, whereas psoriasis is more prevalent in adults than children.

Skin matters

Skin is the largest human organ. It plays an important protective role by providing an interactive boundary between the body and the environment. Skin is repeatedly exposed to ionizing and UV radiation and to potentially toxic dietary and drug metabolites. All these exposures may influence its health and appearance. [1]

Many of these environmental agents and endogenous (inside the body) metabolites are natural oxidants. They can directly or indirectly drive the production of a variety of reactive oxygen species (ROS) or free radicals through a number of physiological processes.[2,3] The surface of the skin is especially sensitive to ROS. Many studies have documented their role in skin aging, the development of inflammatory skin disorders, and carcinogenesis.[1,4,5]

> I developed psoriasis of the scalp due to Calgary's harsh weather conditions. I tried using special shampoos, topical oils and ingested more oils in an attempt to help the psoriasis. It wasn't until I took two capsules of Immuno-Care® per day for one week then one a day for one month that my scalp condition started to improve. I've been taking it for two months and my psoriasis is under control. I believe Immuno-Care® has improved my condition significantly.
>
> *L.F. Calgary, AB*

Simply not superficial

Both eczema and psoriasis can signal more than just cosmetic issues. As a matter of fact, a report in the *Journal of the Royal Society of Medicine* states that eczema is a trigger for other allergic conditions. According to study leader Professor Aziz Sheikh, Chair of the Allergy and Respiratory research group at the University of Edinburgh, "Eczema is a herald condition for individuals who may go on to develop other allergic conditions, such as asthma and allergic rhinitis. The theory is that allergens may be able to cross the skin in people with eczema to cause disease; whereas in people without the condition, the skin is able to act as a barrier."

He added that it is likely that a proportion of individuals have a genetic predisposition to develop eczema, but that environmental factors also play a large part – and it is these factors that are likely to be causing the increase. "Environmental factors include frequency of bathing and use of soaps and detergents. Water use dries up the skin and soaps and detergents degrease the skin. We are using quite a lot of these products from an early age." While soap and water might be part

I am writing you today to let you know something concerning your Immuno-Care® product that you may not be aware of. For most of my life, I have had a very serious problem with cystic acne, the results of which are plainly shown by the scars on my face. The condition has been treated with almost every known medical procedure possible, including massive doses of antibiotics, creams and lotions etc. I am happy to say now that I am completely free of my long term problem for the last 5 months as I have regularly taken Immuno-Care®. I am ecstatic.

K.A., Calgary, AB

of the cause of this skin condition, if left untreated, more serious auto-immune conditions can result.

> I have suffered from varicose eczema for some years, and the doctors seem to think there is no cure. I have used betnovate cream, ichthammol/zinc bandages, coconut oil, and aloe gel at various stages, but none of them have improved the condition. I tried Immuno-Care® and I am pleased to say that there has been a significant improvement in the condition. The itching has decreased and the lesions are decreasing. I would suggest that trials in this area would be useful, as it could eliminate or reduce the use of ointments, (especially steroids which thin the skin long term).
>
> B.G., U.K

Likewise, psoriasis is now linked to many age-related diseases that plague North Americans, like heart disease, high blood pressure and diabetes.

The psoriasis story

Psoriasis turns your skin cells into overachievers. In fact, they mature about five times faster than normal skin cells. But unlike normal skin cells, which naturally slough off, these cells pile up on the skin's surface quickly, like snow on a snow-drift. So why does this happen? What makes these cells go haywire?

Dr. Colby Evans, a psoriasis expert from Texas, says, "We now know that psoriasis is an abnormality or malfunction of the immune system. And, specifically, we know that T-cells, a type of white blood cell, are at the root of it. They are overgrowing and attacking the area of skin where the psoriasis is located. When you biopsy psoriasis and look at it with a microscope, you'll see many T-cells underneath the plaque."

As an inflammatory immune-mediated skin disorder, psoriasis is related to systemic inflammation, which likely contributes to the increased risk of cardiovascular disease in psoriasis patients.[6]

Alike and unlike

The causes of eczema and psoriasis are very different. Eczema is known to be caused by environmental irritants like perfumes, sprays, deodorants, cosmetics, etc. On the other hand, psoriasis is due to genetic factors and not as frequently to environmental factors.

Certain food items also cause flare-ups of eczema. A careful study of which foods cause eczema flare-ups can help keep the condition under control. With psoriasis, there are as yet no such clear indications about foods that may cause flare-ups, though new research connects dietary gluten with psoriasis in some patients. If you suffer with psoriasis and have yet to isolate a cause, talk to your health care provider about testing for celiac disease.[7]

Calming down skin inflammation

Unfortunately, neither eczema nor psoriasis has a final cure. However, proper treatments can help relieve the patient to a large degree. Eczema symptoms are generally less severe but psoriasis symptoms can be very grave in nature and spread all over the body. We also see an association with low levels of antioxidants in the system, and therefore a high degree of oxidative damage to cells and potential DNA damage in psoriasis patients.[8]

Research shows that people with psoriasis may present with low levels of antioxidants and may see a health value when they use antioxidant therapy, particularly as psoriasis is immune-related and shows high inflammatory response. Increasing antioxidants and reducing inflammation with beta-sitosterol may help to alleviate the symptoms of psoriasis.[9]

With their ability to reduce inflammation and balance the immune function, plant sterols and antioxidants can help reduce some of the symptoms associated with these conditions.

---

[1] Sander CS *et al.* Role of oxidative stress and the antioxidant network in cutaneous carcinogenesis. *Int J Dermatol.* 2004 (43):326–335.

[2] Kohen R. Skin antioxidants and their role in aging. *Biomed Pharmacother.* 1999 May :53 (4).

[3] Trouba KJ *et al.* Oxidative stress and its role in skin disease. *Antioxid Redox Signal* 2002 Aug; 4(4).

[4] Briganti S, Picardo M. Antioxidant activity, lipid peroxidation and skin diseases. What's new. *J Eur Acad Dermatol Venereol.* 2003 Nov;17(6).

[5] Okayama Y. Oxidative stress in allergic and inflammatory skin diseases. *Curr Drug Targets Inflamm Allergy.* 2005 Aug; 4(4).

[6] Marzano AV *et al.* Interactions between inflammation and coagulation in autoimmune and immune-mediated skin diseases. *Curr Vasc Pharmacol.* 2012 Jan 20. [Epub ahead of print].

[7] Nagui N *et al.* Estimation of (IgA) anti-gliadin, anti-endomysium and tissue transglutaminase in the serum of patients with psoriasis. *Clin Exp Dermatol.* 2011 Apr;36(3):302-4.

[8] Woźniak A *et al.* Oxidant antioxidant balance in patients with psoriasis. *Med Sci Monit.* 2007;13(1):R 30–R 33.

[9] Young CN *et al.* Reactive Oxygen Species in tumor necrosis factor-alpha-activated primary human keratinocytes: implications for psoriasis and inflammatory skin disease. *J Invest Dermatol.* 2008 (128): 2606–2614.

CHAPTER **THIRTEEN**

Rheumatoid Arthritis

It is probably safe to say that we all know of someone who suffers from rheumatoid arthritis (RA). Yet the disease is not really that well-known outside the circles of people who actually suffer from it. Ask most people and they would not really be able to describe the disease very well. There are other forms of arthritis, but the rheumatoid type has several features that make it different.

One unique part of this disease is that it is symmetrical in pattern; meaning when one knee or hand is involved, usually the other one is also affected. Mostly targeting the wrist joints, finger joints closest to the hand, and knees, RA also targets other parts of the body.

Approximately one percent of North American adults are affected by rheumatoid arthritis. It strikes most often between the ages of 25 and 50 – affecting triple the number of women as men. Studies at the Mayo Clinic show that environmental factors may be to blame. It becomes increasingly important to find ways of supporting the immune system (through diet, supplementation, exercise, relaxation) in order to stack the odds in your favour.

What is rheumatoid arthritis?

While researchers aren't sure yet why it happens, in rheumatoid arthritis the immune system attacks healthy joints, causing inflammation in the lining of the joints. The inflammation can be painful and can lead to permanent damage if the disease is not treated and controlled. RA can also affect other parts of the body, such as the eyes, lungs or heart.

Joint damage can occur even in cases where the pain is not severe. It can happen also in the early stages of the disease. For many people with RA, damage has shown up on X-rays of the hands and feet within two years of the onset of the disease. But it may be too late to fix by the time X-rays discover the problem. One study found that damage got worse more quickly during the first two years, and 75% of all deterioration happened in the first five years.

Severe damage can lead to permanent joint deformity and disability. It can cause so much pain and swelling that one may have difficulty walking, or using hands for routine activities, such as dressing and cooking.

Warning signs of rheumatoid arthritis:
- Morning stiffness that lasts longer than 30 minutes
- Pain in three or more joints at the same time
- Pain in a joint all night long
- Pain in the same joints on both sides of your body, called a symmetrical pattern.

If any warning sign lasts more than two weeks, see your doctor. If your doctor believes that you have RA, it is important to see a rheumatologist right away, so you can begin treatment. RA may start gradually or with a sudden, severe attack with flu-like symptoms. It's important to remember that RA symptoms vary from person to person. In some people, the disease will be mild with periods of activity or joint inflammation (flare-ups) and inactivity (remissions). In other cases, the disease will be continuously active and appear to get worse, or progress, over time. You may feel weak and tired, you may have a fever or lose weight, but joint pain will be the main problem.

Joints affected

One important way to distinguish RA from other forms of arthritis is by the pattern of joint involvement. For example, RA affects the wrist and many of the hand joints but usually not the joints that are closest to the fingernails.

Osteoarthritis, in contrast, affects the joints closest to the fingernails more often than other areas of the hand. In RA, the joints tend to be involved in a symmetrical pattern. That is, if the knuckles on the right hand are inflamed, the knuckles on the left hand are likely to be inflamed as well.

Other joints commonly affected by RA include the elbows, shoulders, neck, jaw, feet, ankles, knees, and hips. Other than the neck, the spine usually is not directly affected by RA.

I want to thank you for recommending Immuno-Care® to me. My rheumatologist put me on prednisone, methotraxate and approved me taking Immuno-Care® I improved rapidly and got off the drugs. I think the Immuno-Care® has helped balance my immune system and helped me fight the RA.

Z.S. Washington

Non-joint involvement

Along with painful, inflamed joints, RA can cause inflammation in other body tissues and organs. In 20% of cases, lumps called 'rheumatoid nodules' develop under the skin, often over bony areas. These occur most often around the elbow, but can also be found elsewhere on the body and even in internal organs.

Occasionally, people with RA will develop inflammation of the membranes that surround the heart and lung or inflammation of the lung tissue itself. Inflammation of tear glands and salivary glands (called sicca syndrome) results in dry eyes and dry mouth. Rarely, RA causes inflammation of the blood vessels (vasculitis), which affects the skin, nerves and other organs.

No one knows for sure what causes RA, although scientists are well on their way to understanding the events that lead to abnormal responses of the body's immune system. We

> I have had RA for some years and I have used the usual NSAIDS and other pain killers but the results were minimal. After trying Immuno-Care®, I can honestly say the pain relief is quite remarkable. Walking used to be my worst experience, as I have RA in the knees hips feet hands and wrists. I am now able to walk without using any aids. I can resume needle work in moderation and even get in and out of buses/cars, and do some household chores. It is truly remarkable. One cannot adequately express pain relief; it is, in part, a feeling of having some joy back in life. The second best part of it all that there are no 'adverse reactions' – it being a natural product and safe to use.
>
> *M.D., BC*

know the disease is not necessarily passed on from generation to generation, but the gene that influences the tendency to have RA is more common in the families of people who have RA. Fortunately, not everyone who inherits this gene will develop the disease.

Canadian scientists are trying to learn why the immune system attacks healthy body tissues. They are also trying to find medicines to help prevent the joint swelling that happens in RA. In fact, *The Arthritis Society* funds many leading-edge research projects that bring vital new insights and lead to new and better treatments for RA.

For example, *The Arthritis Society* is funding a study at the University of Sherbrooke in Quebec, Canada to define markers in the blood that will tell us who will have the mild or serious form of rheumatoid arthritis. At the University of Western Ontario in Canada, a study is looking at a new, very important protein marker for RA. This study will help us understand how the immune system begins to attack joints.

Along with the control of the disease, we must also learn how to regenerate and repair joint tissue, which is the focus of two studies at the Universities of Calgary and Laval: one is examining how genes control the growth of our bones and the other is building frameworks for cells to grow and repair damaged tissue in our joints.

Help yourself

While it may seem counter-intuitive to move painful joints, exercise is just what the doctor orders to reduce pain and prevent further joint damage for those with RA. Other benefits of exercise include weight management, as excess body weight puts more strain on joints. Exercise also helps to strengthen muscles around joints, resulting in less pain.

There are three types of exercises:

- **Range of motion exercises** reduce stiffness and help keep joints moving. A range of motion exercise for your shoulder would be to move your arm in a large circle

- **Strengthening exercises** maintain or increase muscle strength and include lifting weights, yoga, and pilates

- **Endurance exercises** strengthen your heart, give you energy and control your weight. These include walking, swimming and cycling.

Exercise helps lessen symptoms of RA and can make you feel better overall. Appropriate and moderate stretching and strengthening will help relieve the pain and keep the muscles and tendons around the affected joint flexible and strong. Low impact exercises like swimming, walking, water aerobics and stationary bicycling can all reduce pain while maintaining strength, flexibility and cardiovascular function. Of course, you are advised to check with your doctor before beginning an exercise program.

Nutrient matters

As we've seen with several of the autoimmune conditions like eczema and psoriasis, foods and food allergies may also play a role in the genesis and exacerbation of RA.[1,2] If you have RA, keep a food journal to attempt to isolate your possible food triggers, and don't be surprised if your favourite foods are the culprits!

Record what you eat, when you eat it, and how you feel both emotionally and physically. If you note a change in the way you feel – even if it's hours after you eat – make note. Food sensitivity reaction can appear hours or longer after consumption, and may also be the result of meal composition or timing. Although this exercise might seem tedious, it could prove very helpful in isolating your pain triggers.

To the rescue

While foods can be a problem for those with RA, research on phytonutrients suggest they may offer symptom relief. According to a newsletter of *The Arthritis Trust of America*, phytonutrients show potential to alleviate rheumatoid arthritis and other autoimmune disorders:

> "Rheumatoid arthritis is an autoimmune disease. It is postulated that an over-activity of the B-cells causes a release of antibodies, which attach to the synovial tissue of the joints and may destroy the synovium and the joint.
>
> When the antibodies are released, they combine with other antibodies to produce antibody complexes. These may deposit in a joint resulting in the initial recruitment of inflammatory cells, thus precipitating the inflammatory response.
>
> The inflammatory cytokines IL-6 and TNF-alpha have been found in extremely high concentrations in the joints of patients with rheumatoid arthritis.[3] It is known that when macrophages are cultured, IL-6 and TNF-a (which help to start and maintain inflammation) are produced. Strategies targeting IL-6 and IL-6 signaling have been

found to lead to effective treatment of RA and other chronic inflammatory diseases.[4] When cultured with phytonutrients, this production is switched off.

It is also important to note that systemic inflammation hastens the onset of most age-related diseases, and a lesser known fact, individuals with RA have a nearly 40% increased risk of cardiovascular disease.[5]

It is thought that another group of T-helper cells known as TH1(which normally control the immune and inflammatory response) are deficient or damaged in patients with rheumatoid arthritis. Phytonutrients can increase the activity of TH1 cells and decrease the synthesis and release of inflammatory factors. This, therefore, leads to a control of inflammation and a reversal of the immune abnormalities at the disease site.

Existing treatments employ highly toxic drugs to suppress the entire immune response of the body, or to palliate pain and the inflammatory process, without correcting the underlying immune function. Phytonutrients target the immune dysfunction and not the entire immune system. The significant advantage of these phytonutrients is that they are safe, natural and without side effects." [6]

While RA is a painful condition, there is much you can do to find relief: take time to de-stress and heal; exercise regularly; and be sure to create a health-promoting diet, including phytosterols.

Points to note:

Phytonutrients such as those found in Immuno-Care® are very helpful in reducing the inflammation associated with rheumatoid arthritis. Early studies indicated their importance in cholesterol management, but plant sterols in general and beta-sitosterol in particular are now considered potent anti-inflammatory agents with antioxidant analgesic activity.[7]

---

[1] Lidén M *et al.* Self-reported food intolerance and mucosal reactivity after rectal food protein challenge in patients with rheumatoid arthritis. *Scand J Rheumatol.* 2010 Aug;39(4):292-8.

[2] Pattison DJ *et al.* The role of diet in susceptibility to rheumatoid arthritis: a systematic review. *J Rheumatol.* 2004 Jul;31(7):1310-9.

[3] Ishihara K, Hirano T. Il-6 in autoimmune disease and chronic inflammatory proliferative disease. *Cytokine Growth Factor* Rev. 2002 Aug-Oct: 13(4-5):357-68.

[4] Gabay C. Interleukin-6 and chronic inflammation. *Arth Res Ther.* 2006;8 Suppl 2:S3.

[5] Khan F *et al.* The role of endothelial function and its assessment in rheumatiod arthritis. *Nat Rev Rheumatol.* 2010 May; 6(5):253-61.

[6] Gupta MB *et al.* Anti-inflammatory and antipyretic activities of beta-sitosterol. *Planta Med.* 1980 Jun;39(2):157-63.

PART THREE: Lifestyle

CHAPTER **FOURTEEN**

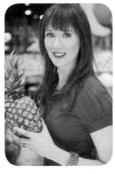 Which Diet is Best?

By: Julie Daniluk, nutritionist, television host and author of the book *Meals That Heal Inflammation*

For years I have been asked, "Which diet should I follow?" You could choose from the Macrobiotic, Diabetic, Paleolithic, Vegan, Vegetarian, South Beach, Specific Carbohydrate, Low Fat, Fruitarian, Atkins, Low Cal, Raw, 100 Mile, Blood Type, The Maker's, Weight Watchers; the list goes on and on. I can understand why people feel so confused about this subject!

Let me tell you my basic food philosophy: there are 6.5 billion different diets for 6.5 billion different people on this planet. I do not believe that there is one generalized diet that is good for everyone. We all come with our own specific medical background that needs our attention so that we can learn what foods we require to be healthy.

I believe in a *Live-it* approach to the food we consume. Dieting suggests a temporary state that you can break off once you have obtained a weight loss goal. You must consider the food you eat by the nutrients it gives you, not just the calories it contains. The cells of your body require a certain amount of macro (proteins, fats and carbohydrates) as well as micronutrients (vitamins, minerals and phytonutrients) in order to function and regenerate. Feeding your body nutrient- dense vegetables and fruit while on a 'diet' only to go back to 'living' on refined carbohydrates and rancid oils is completely counterproductive.

The basic *Live-it*

I believe Michael Pollan's philosophy to: "Eat food, not too much, mostly plants" summarizes a healthy eating model. There is way too much food being consumed in most westernized countries, so the concept of calorie restriction does play a factor in a healthy *Live-it*. I do not believe in actively counting calories, but I do believe it's important to have an awareness of what is high in calories so you can tailor the amount you eat to the amount of activity you participate in. For example, foods such as avocado, coconut, dates, and raw nuts/seeds are all high in macronutrient sugars or fats. These foods are healthy and I'm not advising you avoid them, but you wouldn't want to eat them by the cupful unless you are planning on expending a lot of energy within the next 12 hours.

"Mostly Plants"

After all of the research I have read about diabetes, arthritis, ADHD, heart disease, cancer, weight loss and a host of other diseases, I believe in consuming 10 servings of colourful, organic, fresh vegetables per day. (I do not include corn and white flesh potatoes in this category.) If you have ever tried to eat 10 servings of green, yellow, orange and/or red vegetables in a day, you will know that this does not leave a whole lot of room in your stomach for junk food!

Fruits give you a range of certain phytochemicals that cannot be obtained from other sources, so I believe in eating 2-3 servings of them per day. Besides, they bring so much pleasure! Feeding your emotional self is just as important as feeding your body.

To cook or not to cook?

This is a controversial question in the health food industry. Fresh, organic, raw fruits and vegetables do have the largest amount of nutrient content. They also have the active enzymes that you require to help break down your food. If you do not have Inflammatory Bowel Disease (IBS) and can digest raw whole vegetables and fruit, it is a good way to eat them for the most part. This is particularly true if you live in a warm climate such as the South/West Coast of North America or the Southern States. But eating a lot of cold raw salad, vegetables and fruit is counter-intuitive during the long, cold, damp months of a Canadian winter. It is important to point out that there are certain nutrients that are more bioavailable when they have been cooked so having a variety of cooked and raw foods might be the best balance.

Eating what is available

Not that long ago, many of the diets I mentioned above would simply not be possible, as they require the use of modern day petrochemical transport. I seriously question when someone proposes that we are to only subsist on foods that must be transported from half way around the planet. Don't get me wrong. I enjoy the benefits of organic coconut, olive oil, quinoa, spices and the variety of fresh fruits we have access to throughout the year, but a time may come when we cannot use these products so freely. We need to focus on what we can grow locally to get the nutrients we need to be healthy. Either that or we need to migrate to a location where we can have access to the foods we desire. (Besides, I also strongly believe in supporting our local organic farmers, as they are the backbone to our homegrown health industry.)

Eating meat

A *Live-it* that focuses on high amounts of local vegetation and small amounts of sustainably caught fish, organic poultry and game meat is the best choice for both the environment and your health! That said, there are many people today who are not only unable to digest plant-based proteins, their bodies have built antibodies against them. There is now a technology to determine if you are having an IgE and/or IgG response to food via a blood test. (This is the same technology that is used to match an organ donor to a transplant recipient.) If you consume foods that cause an IgE or IgG response, you are doing more damage than good when you eat them.

If you are unable to eat plant-based proteins such as whole grains, legumes, beans, nuts and seeds because of an intolerance or allergy, you do not have a whole lot of choice when it comes to eating the amount of protein your body requires to build and maintain itself. Eating animal-based proteins may be your only option. If this is the case, it is vital to consume only animals that are raised organically. Animals live at the top of the food chain, therefore, they concentrate any chemicals they are exposed to.

Find out how much protein you actually need in order to be healthy by assessing your physical activity level. When you are growing or training for athletic performance, your needs are higher. They are also higher when you are pregnant or recovering from injury.

Eating like our ancestors

How did our ancestors eat? How did our bodies adapt to the foods that were available? One thing is clear, the *Homo sapiens* that came before us did not have the refined, abundant food products that we consume today. They had to work hard for their food and they earned every calorie. They ate what was available and most likely felt grateful for the plants and animals that they survived on. Waste was not a luxury that could be afforded.

If you lived in what is now known as Canada or Europe 10,000 years ago, you ate a variety of raw and cooked vegetation; cattails, milkweed, dandelion, milk thistle, burdock, nettle, plantain, sumach, mushrooms, leeks, sunchoke, pine needles, hazelnuts, berries, apples and tree sap. You had limited access to honey or salt, but would use it when available. You might collect a bit of wild grain but it was a challenge to have it in a large amount. The predominant protein sources were smaller animals, fowl, insects, fish and seafood if you lived near the ocean. Larger animals were often hunted collectively and every part of their bodies used for food or tools.

Should you return to eating like your ancestors? I think it is a good idea to look back to your roots to find out what your body was designed to thrive on, but it is a challenge to live a strict Paleolithic diet today. You need to take into consideration the region of the world your ancestors came from. What a Paleolithic person would eat in a more tropical region would be very different from a Northern climate. In any case, you would need to spend most of your time hunting, gathering and processing foods and few people have that sort of lifestyle. It would also mean cutting out many wonderful and healthy foods that are available to us from regions we don't live in.

Many of the healthy vegetables and fruit we eat today didn't even exist 10,000 years ago and we would be hard-pressed to recognize their ancestors. Eating a *Live-it* that avoids glutinous grains, refined foods and most dairy products is probably beneficial for most people, but it is important that the Paleolithic diet is not simplified down to eating a heavy, meat-based diet from animals that are factory farmed with a bit of raw vegetation thrown in. Research suggests many of our Paleolithic ancestors were strong, healthy and opportunistic individuals who used a variety of raw and cooked plants and animals to survive.

Phytonutrients, in particular plant sterols, were no doubt a big part of the plants our ancestors ate, and an important part of the foods we eat today. Small but essential components of certain plant membranes, they are found naturally in some vegetable oils, nuts, grains, legumes, fruits and vegetables. In their natural state, sterols are bound to the fibres of plants, and for this reason they are difficult to separate and properly absorb. While seeds are the richest source of plant sterols, refining processes used by the food industry damage and deplete the sterols – which are either removed to make the product completely clear, or destroyed with high-heat processing. The key is to buy unrefined, cold-pressed virgin oils to ensure the healthy sterols are present.

If one chooses to take plant sterol supplements, it is important to take them in an enteric-coated capsule because stomach acids can break sterols down into esters, reducing their effectiveness. It is also important to avoid taking sterols with dairy or animal fat, because the sterols will function to reduce absorption of cholesterol instead of focusing on immune modulation.

Adding plant sterol supplements to your vitamin regime is recommended for most people. Thousands of studies on sterols conducted over 50 years show that they are safe. Multiple sclerosis and diabetes patients and pregnant or nursing mothers should be monitored by a Naturopathic Doctor before considering supplemental use. People with a rare hereditary disease called Sitosterolemia (phytosterolemia) must avoid sterols.

I regularly take Immuno-Care® enteric-coated sterol supplement, and find that I escape most cold and flu rampages. Being a foodie, I am also happy to enjoy sterol-rich gourmet food that both heals the body and satisfies the taste buds!

In summary: eat food, not too much, mostly plants and choose quality supplements.

www.juliedaniluk.com Follow Julie on Twitter, Facebook

Read Julie's new book *Meals That Heal Inflammation* now available across Canada!

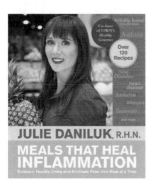

CHAPTER FIFTEEN

Exercise and Health

Simply stated, we want you to feel better, have more energy and perhaps even live longer – and you need look no further than exercise to help you accomplish these goals. The health benefits of regular exercise and physical activity are hard to ignore. From boosting your immune system, to controlling stress, to looking and feeling better, exercise is one of the important daily activities to embrace. And the benefits of exercise are yours for the taking, regardless of your age, sex or physical ability.

Of course, we don't all have to be marathon runners, but many studies are showing the importance of the benefits of regular exercise more than ever before.

Regular exercise boosts immunity

Earlier in the book, we wrote about the many ways to minimize your susceptibility to colds and flu. But did you know that recreational exercisers reported fewer colds once they began running? Moderate exercise has been linked to a positive immune system response and a temporary boost in the production of macrophages, which are the cells that attack bacteria. It is believed that regular, consistent exercise can lead to substantial benefits in immune system health over the long-term.

Energy expenditure through exercise lowers multiple cytokines and pro-inflammatory molecules independently of weight loss. While muscle contraction initially results in a pro-inflammatory state, it paradoxically lowers systemic inflammation. This effect has been observed in dozens of human trials of exercise training in both healthy and unhealthy individuals across many age groups.

Studies show that exercise has the capacity to protect and even enhance the immune response. Researchers have shown that a regular exercise program of brisk walking can bolster many defenses of the immune system, including the antibody response and the natural killer (T-cell) response.

Relatively low levels of aerobic exercise can protect your immune system. Twenty to 30 minutes of brisk walking five days per week is an ideal training program for maintaining a healthy immune response. This is not a lot of exercise and most people should be able to start and maintain this level of activity.

Exercise can also improve your mental wellness, an area that I (Alan) am very interested in and one that I know has helped me greatly. Regular aerobic exercise can help relieve mild to moderate degrees of depression and anxiety. People who exercise also have less loneliness and anger, and are better able to control their own destiny. It is not clear whether exercise boosts the immune system directly or works through a link with the brain and nervous system.

Running toward health and well-being

I (Jack) have a friend who was a clinical psychologist, and he called me one day and asked what drove me to exercising every day, regardless of weather. I live in Calgary, where we often see winter temperatures drop to -30C; regardless, I am out there running in all weather. Even when I travel (which I do a lot), the first thing I pack in my case is my running gear before I think of clean shirts or socks.

I had to stop and think about my friend's question for a moment, and I realized that exercising – especially running – gives me a sense of freedom from the weight of the world we live in. It is like going back to my childhood, running mindlessly, effortlessly and allowing my mind to drift from thought to thought. It also gives me a sense of health and wellness, and I guess it satisfies my urge to be competitive in something I love to do. Although I used to enter many marathons and 10K road races, now I prefer to be out running in the hills or along a river pathway, being one with nature.

I asked my doctor friend why he was interested. He said that he had some patients with whom he was struggling, who suffered severe depression and he wondered if he could interest them in a running program to see if it would help their mood swings and lack of interest in life in general. I know from experience that when you have anxiety and depression, exercise is the last thing you want to do. But I can testify to you that it is one of the best ways to relieve your pain and lighten the load. Although I have had many instances when I have looked out the window and found it hard to get out the door to run, once I made the effort, I have never come back wishing I hadn't run that day. I always come in feeling the joy of having been outside, of running and feeling content and well. I agreed to help him with his plan.

We started off with engaging six of Dr. Kent's patients in a simple walk/run program, and we observed some interesting changes to their clinical depression in short order. The thing to remember with exercise is that it takes a few months to build up the habit, and once that is achieved, it becomes a lifestyle change. The longer you stay with it, the better the result. After six months, Dr. Kent was able to reduce meds and, in some cases, take the patients off their meds with no side effects. It was inspiring and rewarding to see the change that these people made to their mental health by just adding exercise to their daily regimes.

Exercise and cancer

Cancer experts are now in favour of getting their patients up off the couch after typical treatments in order to help reduce the side effects of their therapies. A report done in 2011 by the British Broadcasting Company (BBC) stated some interesting facts, including the assertion that all patients getting cancer treatment be advised to do two and a half hours of physical exercise every week.

Being advised to rest and take it easy after treatment is an outdated view, experts say. Research shows that exercise can reduce the risk of dying from cancer and minimise the side effects of treatment. *Macmillan Cancer Support*, a leading support group based in London, England, published a report stating that of the two million cancer survivors in the UK, around 1.6 million are not physically active enough.

The *British Department of Health Guidelines* recommend that adult cancer patients and cancer survivors undertake 150 minutes of moderately intense physical activity per week. In another report by the *American College of Sports Medicine*, authors also recommend that exercise is safe during and after most types of cancer treatment and suggest that survivors avoid inactivity. Exercise doesn't need to be anything too strenuous: doing the gardening, going for a brisk walk or a swim all count as exercise. Getting active, the report says, can help people overcome the effects of cancer and its treatments, such as fatigue and weight gain: The evidence review shows that physical exercise does not increase fatigue during treatment and can, in fact, boost energy after treatment. It can also lower a patient's chances of getting heart disease and osteoporosis. "Also, doing recommended levels of physical activity may reduce the chance of dying from the disease. It may also help reduce the risk of the cancer coming back." Previous research shows that exercising to the recommended levels can reduce the risk of breast cancer recurring by 40%. For prostate cancer, the risk of dying from the disease is reduced by up to 30%. The risk of bowel cancer patients dying from the disease can be cut by approximately 50% by performing moderate physical activity about six hours per week.

Ciaran Devane, chief executive of *Macmillan Cancer Support*, said physical activity was very important to the survival and recovery process. "Cancer patients would be shocked if they knew just how much of a benefit physical activity could have on their recovery and long-term health. In some cases, exercise reduces [a patient's] chances of having to go through the gruelling ordeal of treatment all over again."

Says Jane Maher, Chief Medical Officer of *Macmillan Cancer Support* and a leading clinical oncologist, "The advice that I would have previously given to one of my patients would have been to 'take it easy.' This has now changed significantly because of the recognition that if physical exercise were a drug, it would be hitting the headlines."

Too much of a good thing

There is also evidence, however, that too much intense exercise can reduce immunity. Marathon runners and endurance athletes often exhibit an increased inflammatory response to injury, as well as immune suppression characterized by frequent bacterial and viral respiratory infections. These outcomes are all the result of high-intensity training. Endurance athletes are often studied because the effects of excessive exercise mimic other stressful events. Excessive physical stress caused by endurance athletics causes tissue damage and in response promotes the release of cortisol and pro-inflammatory cytokines, especially Interleukin-6, DHEA and suppressed immunity.

The synergy: Immuno-Care® and exercise

The plant sterol and antioxidant combination found in Immuno-Care® can also play a part in protecting you during exercise: it has been shown in clinical trials to reduce inflammatory markers such as IL-6. Immuno-Care® reduces oxidative stress and supports the athlete by balancing the all-important immune functions. Athletes currently using Immuno-Care® enjoy much faster muscle recovery time, less lactic acid build-up, and consistent comfort at the end of their exercise periods.

CHAPTER **SIXTEEN**
Immuno-Care®
- Suggested Use

As a dietary supplement, adults can take one Immuno-Care® capsule daily on an empty stomach (30 minutes before eating or at least two hours after eating). It should be taken with water or fruit juice, but not with milk or drinks containing fat.

Research published in the *South African Journal of Science* indicates that a good diet will supply 200 to 300mg of plant sterols per day, and that the amount of plant sterols within the body rapidly diminishes when the diet is deficient in phytonutrients.

Modern food processing methods tend to destroy the phytonutrient content of foods. In addition, the body has difficulty absorbing what phytonutrient content there is left due to the presence of fats in the diet since fats inhibit the absorption of phytonutrients. Immuno-Care® has been formulated to supply the recommended daily intake.

One capsule per day is normally adequate to avoid colds, flu and most allergies, but people with more serious conditions may want to initially double the dose for two weeks, taking one in the morning and one at night.

The body can tolerate high dosages of beta-sitosterol and in one study on cholesterol, participants were given 3 grams per day. The side effects of these high doses were occasional mild constipation, diarrhea or flatulence, and were comparable in frequency to the placebo.

Cautions:

If you are pregnant, nursing, diabetic, taking medication, or under the care of a physician, consult your physician before taking this supplement.

Organ-transplant recipients must not take this supplement.

Keep out of the reach of children.

Ingredients per capsule:

300mg Phytosterols (117mg beta-sitosterol)
50mg Cellasate™
20mg Enzogenol™
30mg Rice Flour

This product is manufactured in Canada a licensed pharmaceutical facility exclusively for Celt Corporation.

©CELT CORPORATION 2012

🍃 Appendix I ————————————————

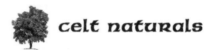

celt naturals

ORIGINAL RESEARCH

Clinical Trial conducted at the University of Guelph,
by the Human Nutraceutical Research Unit

The Supplement Immuno-Care®

Human Nutraceutical Research Unit, J.T. Powell Bldg.
University of Guelph
Guelph, Ontario, Canada N1G 2W1
Tel:(519) 824-4120, ext. 5374
Fax: (519) 823-5247
Website: www.uoguelph.ca/hnru

Maggie Laidlaw, M.Sc., Interim Director, HNRU

———————————————————————————————

This information is provided for educational purposes only and should not be construed as medical advice. Any reader requiring medical advice is strongly advised to consult a licensed health-care professional. Any products mentioned are not intended to diagnose, treat, cure, mitigate or prevent any disease. These statements have not been evaluated by the Food and Drug Administration

Abstract

A randomized, double blind, placebo-controlled clinical trial to determine the effects of Immuno-Care® supplement, (containing plant sterols, pine bark antioxidants and essential fatty acid complex), on specific immune parameters and cardiovascular indices in both men and women with non-food allergies.

The supplement appears to have effect on immune parameters, in particular basophils and Il-6 levels. Given these results this supplement would appear to have the potential to substantially alleviate allergic responses.

The supplement also significantly reduced circulating levels of LDL-cholesterol and increased circulating levels of HDL-cholesterol. There was a significant decrease in the ratio of TC/HDL and in the ratio of LDL/HDL-cholesterol, which corresponds to a decrease in cardiovascular risk, as these ratios are markers for a reduction in the risk for developing atherosclerosis.

Summary of Guelph Trial

This trial was to determine the effects on specific immune parameters and cardiovascular indices of the supplement Immuno-Care® containing plant sterols, pine bark antioxidants and an essential fatty acid complex. The trial was conducted at the University of Guelph as a randomized, double blind, placebo-controlled clinical trial with 20 subjects over 28 days.

RESULTS
Immune Parameters

The effects of the supplement on immune parameters are presented in Table 1. A number of studies support the belief that human basophils play an important role in allergic inflammation. Mast cells and basophils express the high affinity receptor for IgE (FcepsilonRI) and play a central role for IgE-associated immediate hypersensitivity reactions and allergic disorders. During allergic reactions, basophils migrate from the blood compartment to inflammatory sites, where they act as effector cells in concert with eosinophils. Basophils release histamine during inflammation and allergic reactions.

Table 1: *The effects of Immuno-Care® supplementation on specific immune parameters in experimental and placebo groups from day 0 to day 28*

Immune Parameters	Immuno-Care® Day 0	Immuno-Care® Day 28	Immuno-Care® Difference Day 28-Day 0	Control Day 0	Control Day 28	Control % Difference Day 28-Day 0
IgE	472	451	-4.4%	1335	1127	-15.6%
DHEA	6.44	6.44	0 %	4.93	4.77	-3.2%
Cortisol	507	584	15.2%	490	498	1.6%
Cortisol/ DHEA	94.06	108.36	15.2%	160.66	141.44	-12%
IL-6	1.261	0.937	-25.7%	1.318	1.179	10.5%
WBC	7.41	7.24	-2.3%	7.28	7.13	-9.8%
Lymphocyte Count	2.16	2.24	3.7%	2.56	2.60	1.6%
Segmented Neutrophil Count	4.65	4.39	-5.6%	4.11	3.97	-3.4%
Monocytes	0.33	0.34	3.0%	0.35	0.31	-11.4%
Eosinophils	0.24	0.20	-16.7%	0.23	0.20	-13.0%
Basophils	0.23	0.01	- 95.6%**	0.13	0.04	- 69%

** statistically significant, $p < 0.05$

The participants in the treatment group, when compared to the control group, showed a significant reduction in basophil count, while the reduction seen in the control group was non-significant. A reduction in basophil count may indicate a reduction in histamine release.

The immune system also responds to stressors by causing certain immune cells to secrete the pro-inflammatory cytokines, Interleukin-1 (IL-1) and Interleukin-6 (IL-6). These cytokines are both involved in inflammation and IL-6 in particular is thought to worsen the symptoms of autoimmune diseases and fibromyalgia.

Interleukin-6 has been found to act as a growth factor in several tumors and some viruses also use IL-6 to replicate. Interleukin-6 also causes calcium to be released from bone, promoting osteoporosis. We must control the release of these cytokines if we want to enhance immunity and reduce degenerative diseases.

It was noted in the pilot trial that the pro-inflammatory cytokine IL-6 levels showed a substantial reduction in the treated group when compared to the control group. Although the drop in the IL-6 levels in the treatment group was not statistically significant, a larger study with more subjects, over a longer period of time may show significance.

Immuno-Care® has demonstrated that it has an effect on histamine-containing basophil counts and a reduction of IL-6 levels, and consequently may substantially alleviate symptoms associated with airborne allergens, asthma and allergic rhinitis. Further studies are recommended, with a larger patient participation and a longer trial period to investigate other areas of immunological response.

Cardiovascular Parameters

The effects of the supplement on lipid and lipoprotein parameters and cardiovascular indices are illustrated in **Tables 2 and 3**.

Table 2: *The effects of Immuno-Care® on blood lipid parameters in experimental and placebo groups from day 0 to day 28.*

Blood Lipid Parameters (mmol/L)	Immuno-Care® Day 0	Immuno-Care® Day 28	Immuno-Care® Difference Day 28-Day 0	Control Day 0	Control Day 28	Control % Difference Day 28-Day 0
Total Cholesterol	4.36	4.13	-5.3%	4.87	4.91	8.2%
LDL	2.27	1.93	-15.0%**	2.85	2.87	0.7%
HDL	1.63	1.70	4.3%	1.48	1.41	-4.7%
TG	1.00	1.09	9.0%	1.18	1.38	16.9%

** statistically significant, p<0.05

Table 3: *The effects of Immuno-Care® supplementation on specific cardiovascular ratios in experimental and placebo groups from day 0 to day 28.*

Cardio-vascular Parameter Ratios	Immuno-Care® Day 0	Immuno-Care® Day 28	Immuno-Care® Difference Day 28-Day 0	Control Day 0	Control Day 28	Control % Difference Day 28-Day 0
TC/HDL	2.88	2.61	-9.4%**	3.50	3.56	1.7%
LDL/HDL	1.58	1.30	-17.7%**	2.11	2.10	-0.5%
TG/HDL	0.66	0.68	3.0%	0.85	1.02	20.0%

** statistically significant, p<0.05

The specific objective of this portion of the trial was to determine the effects of the supplement Immuno-Care® on blood lipid
parameters. Significant reduction was noted in the overall LDL
levels of the treatment group from day 0 to day 28. Perhaps what
is more interesting is the increase, though not statistically sig-

nificant, in HDL levels compared with a relative decrease in the placebo group.

However it is the ratios of various lipids and lipid proteins rather than the absolute values that are important in assessing cardio-vascular risk, and consequently these ratios were calculated and tabulated.

A significant decrease in the ratio of TC/HDL, and in the ratio of LDL/HDL cholesterol, in the Immuno-Care® group, was noted. A decrease in these ratios corresponds to an associated decrease in the risk of cardiovascular disease (CVD). These ratios are markers for a reduction in the risk of developing atherosclerosis.

Consequently it is our opinion that these results indicate that Immuno-Care® could be very beneficial to the health of hyper-cholesterolemic individuals at risk of developing CVD.

Conclusions

Immuno-Care® and its components appear to have an effect on immune parameters and, in particular, in basophils and possibly IL-6 levels. Given these changes, Immuno-Care® would appear to have the potential to substantially alleviate allergic responses.

Immuno-Care® could also have an effect in auto-immune diseases such as Crohn's disease or rheumatoid arthritis, or in the ability of subjects to resist the common cold virus, although studies on these particular populations would be required to verify possible beneficial effects.

This study verified that Immuno-Care® supplement is effective in reducing circulating levels of LDL-cholesterol and increasing circulating levels of HDL cholesterol.

It is of interest to note that there was a significant decrease in the ratio of TC/HDL, and in the ratio of LDL/HDL cholesterol, in the Immuno-Care® group. A decrease in these ratios corresponds to an associated decrease in cardiovascular disease (CVD) risk, because these ratios are markers for a reduction in the risk of developing atherosclerosis. Consequently, these results would be of considerable benefit to the health of hypercholesterolemic individuals at risk of developing CVD.

Celt Naturals is a division of Celt Corporation, a Canadian company based in Calgary, Alberta Canada. They can be reached at: 1-800-250-8024 © Celt Corporation 2007

🖋 Appendix II

 celt naturals

RESEARCH REVIEW

**Antioxidants, Sterols and Inflammation:
a Natural Approach.**

Alan Fergusson. President, Celt Corporation.

*Presentation to the Functional Medicine Forum, Seattle, Wa., U.S.A.
Immuno-Care®*

This information is provided for educational purposes only and should not be construed as medical advice. Any reader requiring medical advice is strongly advised to consult a licensed health-care professional. Any products mentioned are not intended to diagnose, treat, cure, mitigate or prevent any disease. These statements have not been evaluated by the Food and Drug Administration.

Introduction

Allergies, cardiovascular diseases, fibromyalgia, eczema, asthma and some of the other autoimmune conditions are all diseases involving inflammation, and are frequently treated with pharmaceuticals.

Antioxidants, sterols and inflammation:
a natural approach

1. Antioxidants

Why 'anti' oxidant

Most of you will have heard of antioxidants, but how many of you have wondered why it is necessary to have 'anti' oxidants, when oxygen is essential to life?

The answer lies in the atomic structure of oxygen. As most of you know an atom consists of a nucleus and a series of outside rings, or shells, containing electrons. These rings are particularly stable when they contain specific numbers of electrons, 2, 8, 18, 32 to be precise. Oxygen only has 6 electrons in its outside ring, when it really needs 8 for stability.

So what does it do? It grabs two extra electrons from wherever it can. This leaves an atom or molecule one or two electrons short – it becomes a 'free radical'; then it goes on the hunt to steal electrons from another atom or molecule, and so the process goes on and becomes a chain reaction – creating more 'free radicals' in the process.

Source and effects of free radicals

These free radicals can also be produced by the body's own metabolic process; sometimes the immune system creates them to neutralize viruses and bacteria. However they can also be spawned by environmental factors such as pollution of various sorts, and particularly radiation. If you think you are safe from radiation in this concrete building, then just check your cell, phone! You are also being bombarded by X-rays from your computer.

The problems with free radicals is that they can damage cell membranes through the oxidation of unsaturated fatty acids, and can also be perceived as toxins by the immune system, which can lead to shift towards a Th-2 allergic type response, and all the consequences of an overactive immune system.[1,2,3]

Oxidative stress and inflammation

What is not so well known is that oxidative stress can trigger the production of Il-6, a pro-inflammatory cytokine.[4] Among the factors that normally down regulate this cytokine are estrogen and testosterone, which decline after menopause.

Not surprisingly levels of Il-6 have been found to be elevated in older populations. This age associated rise of Il-6 has been linked to lymphoproliferative disorders, multiple myeloma, osteoporosis and Alzheimer's disease. [5]

Epidemiological studies by the National Institute on Aging have linked elevated Il-6 levels with a high risk of death from cardiovascular disease, and with a high risk of mortality in a population based sample of "healthy" older persons.[6,7] Elevated levels of Il-6 have also been linked to disability onset in older persons, possibly due to a direct effect of Il-6 on muscle atrophy, and/or to the pathophysiologic role played by Il-6 in specific diseases.[8,9]

The bottom line to all this, and one of the major points that I want to make today, is that Il-6 can play a very important role in disease progression, particularly in members of the older population.

Pain and Inflammation

Well, pain is often linked to inflammation; inflammation is

linked to Il-6; Il-6 is linked to oxidative stress [4], so is it possible to alleviate pain through reduction in oxidative stress? – most of you were probably ahead of me at this point!!

Interestingly, in Pubmed there is documented research of cases of pain reduction through the use of antioxidant therapy. These cases involve chronic pancreatitis, prostatitis, asthma, and diabetic neuropathy, - all these involve inflammation and Il-6.[10, 11, 12, 13, 14, 15]

We are going to come back to Il-6 again later, but first, let's take a look at:

2. Sterols

What they are and where they come from

Plant sterols are often referred to as 'plant fats' when, in fact, chemically they are steroidal alcohols – I guess 'steroidal alcohols' does not look too good on the label of a natural health supplement! The name sounds intimidating but if I tell you that they belong to the same chemical class as cholesterol and vitamin D they may sound a little more familiar. They are found in the membranes of most vegetables, fruit and nuts.

They are essential to the body, but like vitamin C, the body cannot synthesize them, they have to be ingested. There are number of sterols in the phytosterol family. The most commonly known are beta-sitosterol, campasterol, brassica-sterol, stigmasterol, and so on. The most important of this class is beta-sitosterol.

For many years, when our diet was mainly plants and vegetables, they were a natural part of our diet.[16,17] However due to the modern processing of food modern diets tend to be deficient in sterols. Furthermore the absorption of the sterols that we do get in our diet is inhibited by the fact that our modern diets generally contain cholesterol, which inhibits the absorption of beta-sitosterol. The dramatic increase in autoimmune and immune related diseases maybe partly related to the absence of plant sterols in our modern diet, as these nutrients help to maintain a balanced immune system.

The main commercial sources of beta-sitosterol are soy[41], sugar cane, canola, and 'the pristine forests'. Allusion to the 'pristine forests' has great marketing potential, but this source is actually the effluent from pulp mills, - not a source that I would choose for my family![48] So in looking at sterols for therapeutic use I would be looking at beta-sitosterol from soy, sugar cane or canola.

The molecular structure of sterols, and particularly beta-sitosterol, is similar to that of other organic compounds produced by the body, in particular cholesterol, vitamin D, and testosterone to name a few – only the side chain varies.

Esters and stanols

You may also hear the terms 'esters' and 'stanols' associated with sterols. Sterol esters are products of sterols and organic acids, where the organic radical replaces the hydroxyl group.

Stanols are hydrogenated sterols, and not familiar to the body. Like hydrogenated oils, we do not know the long-term effects

Sterols in nutrition

Sterols are probably best known for their immune modulating properties.

The body's response to environmental toxins and radiation is a shift to the Th-2 activity, with a consequent loss in Th-1 activity. Sterols can help to modulate this response.[19] This Th-1/Th-2 balance is critical in the development of allergies, eczema and a series of other autoimmune conditions.[20]

Sterols are also reasonably well known for their ability to block the absorption of dietary cholesterol. It is important here to be using 'free sterols', as opposed to esters whose effectiveness declines over a couple of months.[18]

Stanols which are hydrogenated sterols can also block the absorption of cholesterol. However they are not familiar to the body and we do not know their long term effects. Perhaps more importantly they also block the absorption of all sterols, including the beta-sitosterol that is essential to the body.

The advantage of sterols over statins is that while statins block cholesterol production from the liver, (and also inhibit the production of CoQ10), the sterols inhibit the absorption of the dietary cholesterol and leave the liver to control the body's cholesterol levels naturally.[21]

Sterols can also be very helpful to older men suffering from BPH.[22] Not only is this problem a social inconvenience, frequent night time visits to the bath room can result in sleep deprivation, which in turn can have an adverse impact on the immune system, and also result in fatigue and depression.

Sterols and inflammation
Some exciting research is now showing that beta-sitosterol can inhibit the production of the Il-6 that we talked about previously

as being a pro-inflammatory cytokine produced by oxidative stress.[23, 24]

You may recall that epidemiological studies by the National Institute on Ageing have linked elevated levels of IL-6 with increased risk of death from cardiovascular disease.[6,7]

Il-6 has also been linked with disease progression in the older population in a number of diseases, rheumatoid arthritis, multiple myeloma, osteoporosis, Alzheimer's, CVD and mortality in general.[5, 6, 7, 8, 9, 25, 26, 27]

 So Il-6 is certainly a cytokine whose production you would want to minimize. In addition to minimizing Il-6, sterols can also stimulate production of an anti-inflammatory cytokine Il-10.

Il-10 has been associated with inhibition of inflammation,[23, 28, 29, 30] and what is perhaps particularly important, the inhibition of atherosclerotic lesions and blocking atherosclerotic events.[31, 32]

Il-10 has been referred to as an "Immunologic Scalpel" for atherosclerosis, and is under investigation, and in a few cases is at the stage of clinical trials, for therapy for a variety of chronic diseases. These include rheumatoid arthritis, inflammatory bowel disease, psoriasis, and multiple sclerosis.[33, 42]
So, what are the potential applications of:

3. Combined antioxidant / sterol therapy
Probably two of the most prevalent conditions confronting those involved in health care are allergies and fibromyalgia. They both involve oxidative stress and inflammation.[43, 44, 45, 46]

Allergies

A double blind, randomized, placebo controlled trial at the University of Guelph[24] has shown that a patented combination of antioxidants and sterols containing beta-sitosterol, (Immuno-Care), can reduce Il-6 by an average of 35%, and the basophils that release the histamine by an average of 25%. Not surprisingly this antioxidant/ sterol combination has been found in many cases to be effective in alleviating seasonal allergies.

Fibromyalgia

Research by Bagis, Tamer at the University Medical School at Mersin in Turkey[34], and by Fulle, Mecocci at the University of Perugia in Italy[35], found associations between oxidative stress and fibromyalgia, and between oxidative stress and chronic fatigue.

As in many cases fibromyalgia also involves pain and inflammation, it is not surprisingly we are hearing of more and more cases where the symptoms of fibromyalgia and chronic fatigue are being alleviated with a combination of antioxidants and sterols.

Another area of major concern in the healthcare field is the cardiovascular system.

Cholesterol / cardiovascular support

It is well known that "free sterols" can inhibit the absorption of cholesterol. It is important here to focus on the 'free sterols' as opposed to sterol esters which only work for a limited time[18], or stanols that not only inhibit cholesterol absorption, they also inhibit the absorption of the beta-sitosterol that the body needs and cannot make for itself. So it is important to be looking at "free sterols" for cholesterol reduction.

Not only can 'free sterols' inhibit the absorption of cholesterol, they can also reduce the levels of the inflammatory cytokine Il-6, which has been associated with CVD and hypertension.[26, 27]

Il-6 can also be inhibited by antioxidants, as it is triggered by oxidative stress.[4]

A randomized double blind placebo controlled trial of a patented antioxidant/sterol mixture, (Immuno-Care), at the University of Guelph showed an average reduction in LDL of 15%, and an average increase of HDL of 9%. It also showed an average reduction in Il-6 of 35%.

When you couple this with substantial increases in Il-10 [23], with it's association with the prevention of atherosclerotic events [29, 30, 31, 32, 33], you realize that this natural way of providing cardiac support can have many advantages over statins, not least is the fact that you do not interfere with the function of the liver and it's production of CoQ-10. As a bonus it may also reduce C-reactive protein. [47]

BPH

I think that we have already mentioned the use of this combination for BPH [(22)]. I can assure you from personal experience that it is far and away the most effective product on the market for reducing urinary retention, and consequently night time visits to the bathroom that can be a major interruption to a good night's sleep.

The antioxidant component can also help to prevent the development of prostatitis.[12] Urologists in Germany have been using plant sterols to treat enlarged prostates for over twenty years. As side effects, you will also find that your patients will have lower cholesterol levels, and get fewer flu's and colds!

Generally speaking this antioxidant/sterol combination can be very helpful in alleviating the symptoms of most autoimmune disease such as eczema, psoriasis, rheumatoid arthritis, asthma, etc.[42]

In fact there is one senior member of BioGenesis who can attest to its effectiveness in alleviating symptoms of asthma.[42]

4. Why Immuno-Care?
There are several reasons for using Immuno-Care.

First, it is very important to reduce the oxidative stress within the body. Immuno-Care contains Enzogenol, a very powerful broad spectrum antioxidant derived from the bark of selected pine trees, which contains over 2,000 different flavonoids - probably the most comprehensive complex of natural antioxidants yet discovered.

The patented extraction process, developed by the University of Canterbury in New Zealand, uses only pure water, which ensures that significant groups of antioxidants are harvested, and not lost as in the conventional solvent based process.
Secondly, in order to inhibit Il-6 and promote Il-10, Immuno-Care incorporates "free sterols", that is sterols free of the esters or stanols, and the sterols are derived from soy, and not wood pulp

Thirdly is the inclusion of a proprietary blend of amino acids, enzymes and peptides designed to facilitate the absorption and retention of the sterols and antioxidants.

As far as I know no other manufacture of sterol products has paid attention to the issue of absorption and retention of the sterols. And this is important as sterols normally are difficult to absorb and only stay in the body for a short period of time.

Fourthly, I am sure that some of you are waiting to ask me if sterols are actually steroidal alcohols, then what happens to them when they hit stomach acid ?

That is a very good question, and the question is equally relevant to the antioxidants, as they also have hydroxyl groups in their molecular structure. The answer is that they would turn into sterol esters, which you may remember only work for a limited period of time.

So, how do we prevent that? Well, as far as I know, Immuno-Care contains the only encapsulated sterols that are enteric coated, so that they pass through the stomach acids and dissolve in the alkaline environment of the small intestine. This ensures that the sterols and antioxidants pass through the stomach without being destroyed and also facilitates the absorption and retention of both the sterols and the antioxidants.

This is really a technical achievement. As far as I know, we are the only company that enteric coats two-piece vegetable capsules containing sterols to ensure the absorption, probably because it is a very difficult process with a large wastage.

The spraying process is a very difficult, too much and the whole batch turns into a soggy mass, too little and the enteric coating is not effective. The drying process is again critical, too slow and the capsules dissolve and you are left with a soggy mess again, too fast and the capsules crack during the bottling process. There is a very large wastage.

5. The last word

As a final word, one of the things that really amazed me when I first started this journey into the natural health field was when I discovered that people with multiple personalities showed different symptoms in different personalities.

There is a classic case mentioned by Depak Chopra in his book *Quantum Healing* where this man is diabetic in one personality, but when he changes personality his blood sugars return to normal. In another personality he is allergic to orange juice and will burst out in hives. But when he changes personality all the hives disappear.

Another case was a patient of Bernie Siegel, who had to sleep with three pairs of glasses by her bedside, as she was never quite sure which personality she would wake up in.

This tells me the power of the mind – and if you do not believe me, just think about the placebo effect! The mind is incredibly powerful, and the biggest threat to our immune system comes from stress. There is no simple answer to this, but laughter, good friends, exercise and sleep can help.

It is important to find time for relaxation and peace, to find your own path up the mountain, whether this is through music, running, skiing, or particular religious practices. The important thing is to climb the mountain. [49]

Celt Naturals is a division of Celt Corporation, a Canadian company based in Calgary, Alberta, Canada. They can be reached at 1-800-250-8024. © Celt Corporation 2012

---

[1] Free Radicals, Antioxidants and Nutrition. Fang, Yang et al. Dept. Biochem. and Molecular Biol., Beijing Inst. of Radiation Beijing, China. Nutrition 2002, Oct. 18(10)

[2] Antioxidants, Oxidative Damage and Oxygen Deprivation Stress. Blokhina, Vrolainen et al. Dept Bioscience, Helsinki University, Helsinki, Finland. Annals of Botany 2003;91 Spec No 179-94

[3] Antioxidants to Slow Aging, Facts and Perspectives. Bonnrfoy, Drai el. Service de Medicine Geriatrique, Lyon. France. Presse Medicale, (France), 2002 Jul 31(25):1174-84

[4] Serum Antioxidants, Inflammation, and Total Mortality in Older Women. Walston, Xue et al. School of Medicine, John Hopkins University. U.S.A., Am. Jnl. Epidem 2006, 163(1)18-26.

[5] Age Associated Interleukin-6 Expression and Late Life Diseases. Ershler, Keller. Inst. For Advanced Studies in Aging and Geriatric Med, Washington, DC., U.S.A. Annual Rev of Medicine, 2000;51:245-70.

[6] Cardiovascular Disease, Interleukin-6 and Risk of Mortality in Older Women. Volpato, Guralnik et al. National Institute on Aging, Bethesda, U.S.A. Circulation 2001 Feb 103(7)

[7] Associations of Elevated Interleukin-6 and C-Reactive Protein levels with Mortality in the Elderly. Harris, Ferrucci et al. Nat. Inst. On Aging, Bethesda. U.S.A., Am. Jnl. Med. 1999 May;106(5):506-12.

[8] Serum Il-6 Level and Development of Disability in Older Persons. Ferrucci, Harris et al. INRCA, Florence, Italy. Jnl. Am Geriatric Soc. 1999 Jun:47(6):639-46.

[9] Dietary Carotenoids and Risk of Coronary Artery Disease in Women. Osganian, Meir et al. Harvard School of Public Health. Am. Jnl. CL. Nutr. 2003 June. Vol 77(6) 1390-99.

[10] Combined Antioxidant Therapy Reduces Pain in Chronic Pancreatitis. Kirk, White, et al. Royal Victoria Hosp, Belfast, U.K., Jnl. Gastrointest. Surg. 2006 Apr.:10(4):499-503.

[11] Use of Antioxidants in Chronic Pancreatitis. Castano, Paz et al. Valdecilla University Hosp. Spain. Revista Espanola Enfermedades, Digestivas 2000 June;92(6):375-85.

[12] Quercetin In Men with Category 3 Prostatitis. Shoskes, Zeitlin et al. Harbor-UCLA Med Centre, UCLA., Ca., U.S.A., Urology, Dec 1999, Vol 54(6) 960-963

[13] ALA Improves Symptoms of Diabetic Neuropathy. Dyck, Low, Litchy. Mayo Clinic. Diabetes Care, March 2003

[14] Pycnogenol in the Management of Asthma. Hosseini, Pishnamazi et al. School of Medicine, University of Arizona. Med. Food 2001 Winter 4(4):210-209

[15] Plasma C-Reactive Protein Concentrations: Influence of Antioxidant Supplementation. Block, Jensen, et al. Dept. Nutritional Sc. Univ. Cal. (Berkeley). U.A.A. Jnl. AM. Col Nutr vol 23, (2) 141-7.

[16] Importance of Sitosterol in Human and Animal Nutrition. Pegel. University of Natal, S. African Jnl. Sc. S.A. 1997. vol 93 , 263-7.

[17] The Garden of Eden – Plant Based Diets. Jenkins, Kendall et al. St Michael's Hospital, Toronto. Comp. Biochem. Physiol A Integr Pysiol. 2003, Sep;136

[18] Comparison of Plant Sterol and Stanol Esters on Lipid Metabolism. O''Neil, Brynes et al. Faculty of Medicine, Imperial College London.U.K., Nutr. Metab. Cardiovasc. Dis., 2004 June 14(3):133-42

[19] Flow Cytometric Analysis of the Th1-Th2 Balance. Breytenbach, Clark et al. Dept Medical Biol. Univ Stellenbosch, Capetown, S.A., Cell Biol Intl.2001;25(1):43-9.

[20] Immune Response in Healthy and Allergic Individuals Characterized by Balance between Allergen Specific Th1 and Th2 cells. Akdis, Verhagen et al. Swiss Institute of Allergy and Asthma Research. Davos, Switzerland. Jnl. Exp Med. 2004 June 199(11):1567-75

[21] Efficacy and Safety of Plant Stanols and Sterols in the Management of Blood Cholesterol Levels. Katan, Grundy et al. Mayo Clinic Proceedings. 2003:78:965-78

[22] A Multicentric, Placebo-controlled, Double-blind, Trial of Beta-Sitosterol for BPH. Klippel, Hiltl et al., Dept Urol., Academic Hospital, Germany. Br. Jnl. Urol 1997 Sep;80(3):427-32

[23] Antiatherogenic Effects of Plant Sterols Associated with Inhibition of Proinflamatory Cytokine Production. Nashed, Yeganeh et al. St Boniface Hospital and the University of Manitoba, Winnipeg, Man.,Canada. Am. Soc. Nutr. Sc, Jnl. Nutr 2005 Oct 135:2438-2444

[24] Pilot Study on the Supplement Immuno-Care. Laidlaw. Human Nutraceutical Research Unit. University of Guelph, Ontario, Canada.

[25] Interleukin-6 and Chronic Inflammation. Gabay, C. Div Rheum., University Hospital, Geneva. Switzerland. Arthritis Res. Ther 2006;8 Supp2:S 3.

[26] Associations of elevated Il-6 and C-reactive Protein levels with Mortality in the Elderly. Harris, Ferrucci et al. National Institute on Aging, Bethesda. U.S.A. Am.J.Med 1999 May;106(5):506-12.

[27] Inflammation, Obesity, Stress and Coronary Heart Disease: Is Il-6 the Link? Yudkin, Kumari et al. University College Medical School, London. U.K., Atherosclerosis 2000 Feb;148(2):209-14

[28] Aging, Longevity, Inflammation and Cancer. Caruso, Lio et al. Dept. Immunol., Univ. Palermo, Italy. Ann. N. Y. Acad. Sc. 2004, vol.1028

[29] Immunoregulatory Role of Interleukin 10 in Inflammatory Bowel Disease. Schreiber, Heinig et al. Dept. Med.. Univ. Hamburg, Germany. Gasteroenterology 1995 May;108(5):1434-44

[30] Essential Role of Il-10 in the Function of T-cells Inhibiting Intestinal Inflammation. Asseman, Mauze et al. Radcliffe Hosp. Univ. Oxford, U.K., and DNAX Res. Inst. Mol. Biol., Palo Alto, Ca. U.S.A. Jnl. Exp. Med. Oct 1999. Vol 190(7)

[31] Protective Role of Il-10 in Atherosclerosis. Mallet, Besnard et al. Inst. Nat. Sante Res. Med, Paris, France. Circulation Res.1999 Oct. 15;85(8) .

[32] Il-10 Blocks Atherosclerotic Events in Vitro and In Vivo. Oslund, Hendrick et al. UCLA Mol. Biol. Inst. Los Angeles, Ca. U.S.A. Arteriosclerosis, Thrombosis, and Vascular Biol. 1999(19)

[33] Il-10: An "Immunologic Scalpel" for Arterosclosis. Terkeltaub R.A., San Diego VA Med Centre. Arteriosclerosis, Thrombosis and Vascular Biology 1999 vol 19 (12).

[34] Free Radicals and Antioxidants in Primary Fibromyalgia. Bagis, Tamer et al. Univ. Med .Schl., Mersin, Turkey. Rheumatology International. 2005 Vol 25 (3).

[35] Specific Oxidative Alterations in Vastus Lateralis Muscle in CFS Patients. Fulle, Mecocci et al., Univ Perugia, Italy. Free Radic. Biol. 2000Dec. 15; 29 (12):1252-9.

[36] Reactive Oxygen Intermediates Stimulate Il-6 Production in Human Bronchial Epithelial Cells. Yoshida, Maruyama et al., Toyama Medical Univ., Japan. Am. Jnl. Physiol. Lung Cell. Physiol. June 1999, 276(6).

[37] Ultraviolet Light Induces Increased Circulating Il-6 in Humans. Urbanski, Schwarz et al. Univ of Vienna and Boltzmann Inst., Vienna, Austria. Jnl. Invest. Derm., 1990 vol 94, 808-811.

[38] Il-10 Inhibits Vascular Smooth Muscle Cell Activation in Vitro and in Vivo. Mazighi, Pelle et al., Inst. Nat Health and Med. Res. Central University Hosp. Paris, France. A. J. Physiol. Heart Circ Physiol April 2004, 287;H866-71.

[39] Il-10 Required for Protection Against Atherosclerosis. Potteaux, Esposito, et al.INSERM, Hospital Lariboisiere,Paris, France. Arth. Throm.Vasc Biol. 2004:24:1474

[40] Il-10:An Update on it's Relevance to Cardiovascular Risk. Girnt, Kohler. Dept Med., Univ. Saarland, Germany. Nephrology Dialysis Transplantation 2003, vol 18 (10), 1976-79.

[41] The Evidence for Soybean Products as Cancer Preventative Agents. Kennedy A.R., Dept Oncol., Univ. Penn. Med. Sch. J. Nutr 1996 Feb;126(2).

[41] Treatment of Psoriasis with Il-10. Reich, Bruck et al. Dept. Derm. Gottingen and Tubingen Univs. Germany. Jnl. Investig. Derm. 1998 Vol 3(6).

[43] Oxidative Stress in Allergic Respiratory Diseases. Russell, Bowler, et al. Nat. Jewish Med. Centre, Denver. Jnl. Allergy Clin. Immunol. 2002. Vol. 110(3).

[44] Oxidative Stress Generated by Intrinsic Pollen. Boldogh, Bacsi, et al. Univ Texas. Jnl. Allergy Immunol. 2004. vol. 113(2)Sup 1.

[45] Oxidative Stress in Allergic and Inflammatory Skin Diseases. Okayama Y. Res. Centre Allergy and Immunology. Yokohama, Japan. Current Drug Targets – Inflammation and Allergy, 2005 vol. 4(4).

[46] Ultrafine Particulate Pollutants Induce Oxidative Stress and Mitochondrial Damage. Li, Sioutas, et al. Dept Med. UCLA., Los Angeles, Ca. Enviro. Health Perspectives 2003 April; 111(4).

[47] Reduced Calorie Orange Juice Beverage with Plant Sterols Lowers C-reactive Protein. Devaraj, Autret et al. Laboratory for Atherosclerosis and Metabolic Res. UCLA at Davis, Ca. Am. J. Clin. Nutr. 2006 Oct;84(4).

[48] Technologies for Reducing Dioxin in the Manufacture of Bleached Wood Pulp. U.S. Congress, Office of Technology Assessment. OTA-BP-O-54 (Washington, DC: U.S. Government Printing Office, May 1989. Library of Congress Cat 89-600719.

[49] "Peace, Love and Healing". Bernie Siegel, M.D., Harper and Row. ISBN 0-06-091705-9. Lib. Congr. 89-82587.

For more information please call:
CELT NATURALS at
1-800-250-8024

🍃 Notes ────────────────────────────